W

Nurses! Test Yourself in Clinical Skills

Nurses! Test Yourself in ...

Visit www.mcgraw-hill.co.uk/openup/testyourself for further information and sample chapters from other books in the series.

Nurses! Test Yourself in Clinical Skills

Edited by Marian Traynor

JET LIBRARY

Open University Press

Open University Press
McGraw-Hill Education
McGraw-Hill House
Shoppenhangers Road
Maidenhead
Berkshire
England
SL6 2QL

email: enquiries@openup.co.uk
world wide web: www.openup.co.uk

and Two Penn Plaza, New York, NY 10121–2289, USA

First published 2012

Copyright © Marian Traynor, 2012

A catalogue record of this book is available from the British Library

ISBN-13: 978-0-33-524483-6 (pb)
ISBN-10: 0-33-524483-1 (pb)
eISBN: 978-0-33-524484-3

Library of Congress Cataloging-in-Publication Data
CIP data applied for

Typesetting and e-book compilations by
RefineCatch Limited, Bungay, Suffolk
Printed and bound in the UK at Bell & Bain Ltd, Glasgow.

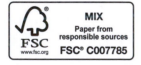

MIX
Paper from
responsible sources
FSC® C007785

The *McGraw·Hill* Companies

Dedicated to Anne Gallagher and Lorna Martin. Thank you both!

Nursing is one of the most difficult of acts. Compassion may provide the motive but knowledge is our only working power. (Mary Adelaide Nutting 1925)

Contents

About the authors

Editor

Dr Marian Traynor is an Assistant Director of Education and Discipline Lead for Clinical Learning, Simulation, Research and Development in the School of Nursing and Midwifery at Queen's University, Belfast. She teaches undergraduate students of nursing in the adult branch and has a special interest in Objective Structured Clinical Examination (OSCE), clinical assessment and simulation.

Contributors

Mrs Gillian Trinick is a Nurse Lecturer in the School of Nursing and Midwifery at Queen's University, Belfast. She teaches undergraduate students of nursing in the adult and mental health branches and has a special interest in diabetes, neurology and haematology oncology nursing. She is involved in facilitating learning through the use of Simulation Practice.

Mrs Frances Auld is a Nurse Lecturer in the School of Nursing and Midwifery at Queen's University, Belfast. She teaches undergraduate students of nursing in the adult branch and has a special interest in clinical skills. She is involved in facilitating learning through the use of Simulation Practice.

Mrs Beverly McClean is a Nurse Lecturer in the School of Nursing and Midwifery at Queen's University, Belfast. She teaches undergraduate students of nursing in the adult branch and has a special interest in nutrition. She is involved in facilitating learning through the use of Simulation Practice.

Mr Edmund Shields is a Nurse Lecturer in the School of Nursing and Midwifery at Queen's University, Belfast. He teaches undergraduate students of nursing in the adult branch and has a special interest in respiratory nursing and nursing research.

Using this book

Welcome to *Nurses! Test Yourself in Clinical Skills*. We hope you will find this an invaluable tool throughout your clinical skills courses and beyond!

This book is designed to be used as a revision aid that you can use with your main textbook. Each chapter is designed for stand-alone revision, meaning that you need not read from the beginning to benefit from the book.

Each chapter begins with a brief introduction covering the main points of the topic and directing you to some useful resources. The chapter progresses providing you with different types of questions that help you test your knowledge of the area. These are:

- *Labelling Exercise:* identify the different elements on the diagram. A list of terms is given to assist you.
- *True or False:* identify if the statement is true or false.
- *Multiple Choice*: identify which of four answers is correct.
- *Fill in the Blanks*: fill in the blanks to complete the statement.
- *Match the Terms*: identify which term matches which statement.
- *Chart Exercises*: complete the chart.

The questions have been designed to be slightly more challenging in each section. Do not ignore a question type just because you are not examined in that way, because the answer will contain useful information that could easily be examined in an alternative question format. Answers are provided in each chapter with detailed explanations – this is to help you with revision but can also be used as a learning aid.

We have suggested some useful textbooks and other resources that may be used to support your recommended text, but be aware that they should not replace the core reading for your course.

At the back of the book there is an appendix where you will find a glossary, and at the front a list of directional terms and a list of common prefixes and suffixes commonly used in clinical practice.

We hope that you enjoy using this book and that you find it a convenient and useful tool throughout your studies!

List of abbreviations

ABCDE	Airway, Breathing, Circulation, Disability and Exposure	HSE	Health and Safety Executive
ANTT	aseptic non-touch technique	ICU	Intensive Care Unit
		IFCC	International Federation of Clinical Chemists
AVPU	Alert; Responds to vocal stimuli; Responds to painful stimuli; Unresponsive to all stimuli	IHI	Institute for Healthcare Improvement
		IM	intramuscular
		IV	Intravenous Therapy
		LVF	Left Ventricular Failure
BAPEN	British Association for Parenteral and Enteral Nutrition	MHOR	Manual Handling Operations Regulations
		MI	Myocardial Infarction
BMI	Body Mass Index	mmHg	millimetres of mercury
BNF	British National Formulary	MRSA	Methicillin Resistant *Staphylococcus Aureus*
CNS	central nervous system		
COPD	chronic obstructive pulmonary disease	MUST	Malnutrition Universal Screening Tool
CPR	cardiopulmonary resuscitation	NG	nasogastric
		NGASR	Nurse's Global Assessment of Suicide Risk
CRT	capillary refill time		
CSCG	Clinical and Social Care Governance	NHS	National Health Service
CSU	catheter specimen of urine	NICE	National Institute for Health and Clinical Excellence
DPI	dry powder inhaler		
DVLA	Driver Vehicle Licensing Authority		
		NMC	Nursing and Midwifery Council
ECG	electrocardiogram		
EWS	early warning score	NPSA	National Patient Safety Agency
G	gauge		
GCS	Glasgow Coma Scale	NQB	National Quality Board
GMC	General Medical Council	PEF	Peak Expiratory Flow
HCAI	HealthCare-Associated Infection	PEG	Percutaneous Endoscopic Gastrostomy

PEWS	Physiological Early Warning Signs	**SBAR**	Situation, Background, Assessment and Recommendation
pMDI	pressured Metered Dose Inhaler	**SC**	subcutaneous (injection)
PPE	personal protective equipment	**SoPs**	Standard operating Procedures
RAS	Reticular Activating System	**UTI**	Urinary Tract Infection
		WHO	World Health Organization

Guide to useful resources

Websites

Asthma UK
www.asthma.org.uk/health_professionals/index.html

British Association for Parenteral and Enteral Nutrition (BAPEN)
www.bapen.org.uk

Department of Health:
http://www.dh.gov.uk

Department of Health Competencies for recognising and responding to acutely ill patients in hospital
http://www.dh.gov.uk/en/Publicationsandstatistics/Publications/PublicationsPolicyAndGuidance/DH_096989

Health and Safety Executive Manual handling assessment charts
www.hse.gov.uk/pubns/indg383.pdf

Health and Safety Executive Short guide to regulations and risk assessment
www.hse.gov.uk/pubns/indg143.pdf

Institute for Healthcare Improvement
www.ihi.org

Monthly Index Medical Services (MIMS)
www.mims.co.uk

National Back Exchange (NBE)
http://www.nationalbackexchange.org.uk

National Institute for Health and Clinical Excellence (NICE)
www.nice.org.uk

National Patient Safety Agency (NPSA)
www.npsa.nhs.uk

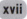

NHS Diabetes
www.diabetes.nhs.uk/safe_use_of_insulin/elearning_course/

Nursing Times – Respiratory nursing
www.nursingtimes.net/section2.aspx?navcode=1335

World Health Organization
http://www.who.int

Books, journals and other resources

Advanced Life Support (6th edition)
J. Nolan, J. Soar and A. Lockey
Published by Resuscitation Council (UK), 2011

Essential Nursing Skills (3rd edition)
M. Nicol, C. Bavin, P. Cronin and K. Rawlings-Anderson
Published by Mosby, 2008

Head Injury: Triage, Assessment, Investigation and Early Management of Head Injury in Infants, Children and Adults
National Institute for Health and Clinical Excellence (NICE)
Published by NICE, 2007
Available at: http://guidance.nice.org.uk/CG56

Nurses! Test Yourself in Anatomy and Physiology
K.M.A Rogers and W.N. Scott
Published by McGraw-Hill, 2011

Nurses! Test Yourself in Essential Calculation Skills
K.M.A Rogers and W.N. Scott
Published by McGraw-Hill, 2011

Nurses! Test Yourself in Pathophysiology
K.M.A Rogers and W.N. Scott
Published by McGraw-Hill, 2011

Mader's Understanding Human Anatomy and Physiology (7th edition)
S. Longenbaker
Published by McGraw-Hill, 2011

Standards for Medicines Management
Nursing and Midwifery Council
Published by NMC, 2007
Available at: www.nmc-uk.org

The Royal Marsden Hospital Manual of Clinical Nursing Procedures
(8th edition)
L. Dougherty and S.E. Lister (eds)
Published by Wiley-Blackwell, 2011

Directional terms

Abduct   move away from the midline of the body; the opposite of adduct

Adduct   movement towards the midline of the body; the opposite of abduct

Anterior   front-facing or ventral; opposite of posterior or dorsal

Contralateral   on opposite side; opposite of ipsilateral

Distal   far away from point of origin; the opposite of proximal

Dorsal   to the back or posterior of; opposite of ventral or anterior

Inferior   lower or beneath; opposite to superior

Ipsilateral   on same side; opposite to contralateral

Lateral   referring to the side, away from the midline; opposite of medial

Medial   towards the middle; opposite of lateral

Posterior   back or dorsal; opposite of anterior or ventral

Proximal   nearest to the centre of the body; opposite of distal

Superior   above or higher; opposite of inferior

Ventral   referring to front or anterior; opposite of dorsal or posterior

The table below summarizes how these terms match up.

Direction	Opposite term
Abduct	Adduct
Anterior/ventral	Posterior/dorsal
Contralateral	Ipsilateral
Distal	Proximal
Inferior	Superior
Lateral	Medial

Common prefixes, suffixes and roots

Prefix/suffix/root	Definition	Example
a-/an-	deficiency, lack of	anuria = decrease or absence of urine production
-aemia	of the blood	ischaemia = decreased blood supply
angio-	vessel	angiogenesis = growth of new vessels
brady-	slow	bradykinesia = slow movements
broncho-	bronchus	bronchitis = inflammation of the bronchus
card-	heart	cardiology = study of the heart
chole-	bile or gall bladder	cholecystitis = inflammation of gall bladder
cyto-	cell	cytology = study of cells
derm-	skin	dermatology = study of the skin
dys-	difficult	dysphagia = difficulty swallowing
-ema	swelling	oedema = abnormal accumulation of tissue fluid
entero-	Intestine	enteritis = inflammation of the intestinal tract
erythro-	red	erthyropenia = deficiency of red blood cells
gast-	stomach	gastritis = inflammation of stomach lining
-globin	protein	haemoglobin = iron-containing protein in the blood
haem-/haemo-	blood	haemocyte = a blood cell (especially red blood cell)
hepat-	liver	hepatitis = inflammation of the liver

-hydr-	water	*rehydrate = replenish body fluids*
-itis	inflammation	*bronchitis = inflammation of the bronchus*
-kinesia	movement, motion	*bradykinesia = slow movements*
leuco-	white	*leucopenia = deficiency of white blood cells*
lymph-	lymph tissue/ vessels	*lymphoedema = fluid retention in lymphatic system*
lyso-/-lysis	breaking down	*hydrolysis = breaking down molecule with water*
myo-	muscle	*myocardium = cardiac muscle*
nephro-	kidney	*nephritis = inflammation of the kidneys*
neuro-	nerve	*neurology = study of the nerves*
-ology	study of	*dermatology = study of the skin*
-oma	tumour	*lymphoma = tumour of the lymph tissue*
-opthth-	eye	*ophthalmology = study of the eyes*
os-/osteo-	bone	*osteology = study of bones*
path-	disease	*pathology = study of disease*
-penia-	deficiency of	*leucopenia = deficiency of white blood cells*
pneumo-	air/lungs	*pneumonitis = inflammation of lung tissue*
tachy-	excessively fast	*tachycardia = excessive heart rate*
-tox-	poison	*toxicology = study of poisons*
-uria	urine	*haematuria = blood in the urine*
vaso-	vessel	*vasoconstriction = narrowing of vessels*

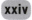

1 Infection control

INTRODUCTION

Modern technology within the healthcare setting has brought many advantages; despite this, however, many patients still suffer and die from healthcare-associated infections (HCAIs). Globally, there is much concern regarding the rise of HCAIs and the challenges they present. Effective high-quality practices that are reliable and specific to the context of care must be adhered to by all healthcare professionals in an attempt to minimize the increased risk of infection. Awareness and assessment of the environment of care and the potential for infection within it must be constantly reviewed by individual practitioners to effectively identify and reduce any risks to patient and others.

Preventative measures against the spread of infection are one of the key skills required by every nurse. In recent years, there have been many changes in practice regarding infection control measures and it is the responsibility of each individual nurse to update his or her knowledge and skills in this area.

Useful resources

Department of Health:
http://www.dh.gov.uk

Institute for Health Improvement:
http://www.ihi.org

National Institute for Health and Clinical Excellence (NICE):
http://www.nice.org.uk

National Patient Safety Agency:
http://www.npsa.nhs.uk

World Health Organization:
http://www.who.int

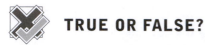 **TRUE OR FALSE?**

Are the following statements true or false?

 Bacteria grow faster under gloved than ungloved hands.

 Surgical site infections contribute to nosocomial infections.

 When washing hands, using a nailbrush helps to remove bacteria and leaves hands cleaner.

 Gloves may be washed and reused for the same patient.

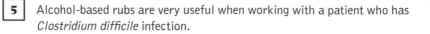 Alcohol-based rubs are very useful when working with a patient who has *Clostridium difficile* infection.

 Artificial nails are acceptable if kept clean.

7 Hands should be wetted under running water and liquid soap applied before rubbing together vigorously.

8 If disposable towels are unavailable, it is acceptable to use the patient's towel to dry your hands.

The complete process of hand washing should take no less than 40 seconds.

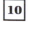 The non-touch technique can be incorporated as part of a clean procedure.

 When using sterile gloves, hand washing is not crucial.

MULTIPLE CHOICE

Identify one correct answer for each of the following.

12 The most common way of spreading infection in a healthcare environment is via:

a) overuse of antibiotics

b) patient isolation

c) hands of healthcare staff

d) toilet seats

13 The choice of personal protective equipment (PPE) is made by:

a) the nurse after assessing the situation

b) the doctor in charge of the patient

c) the infection control team

d) the ward manager

14 Isolation nursing is:

a) intended to prevent the spread of infection to patients and others

b) wearing personal protective clothing at all times

c) wearing gloves and aprons during all patient contact

d) ensuring no visitors are allowed

15 Gloves should be worn:

a) for handling items contaminated with blood

b) when feeding a patient with MRSA

c) when administering oral medications

d) when charting the observations of a patient in isolation

16 Sterile gloves should be used when:

a) carrying out urinary catheter care

b) inserting a urinary catheter

c) erecting intravenous fluids

d) performing venepuncture

17 Which of the following contributes to the prevention of oro-faecal contamination?

a) drinking only bottled water

b) disposable rubbish bags

c) provision of hot water, soap, and towels

d) non-sterile gloves

18 'Superbugs' are:

a) any infection acquired in the healthcare environment

b) pathogens that have become resistant to treatment

c) cockroaches found in healthcare environments

d) specific viral infections

19 MRSA stands for:

a) microorganisms resistant to specific antibiotics

b) methicillin-resistant *Staphylococcus aureus*

c) micro-resistant *Staphylococcus aureus*

d) methicillin-reactive *Staphylococcus aureus*

20 A care bundle is:

a) a checklist

b) a small essential set of evidence-based practices

c) a parcel of local policies

d) a set of patient care procedures

21 The aseptic non-touch technique involves the use of:

a) face masks

b) sterile gloves

c) dressing pack

d) sodium chloride

22 An aseptic technique should be carried out for procedures such as:

a) surgical wound dressing

b) urinary catheter care

c) blood glucose monitoring

d) administration of eye drops

FILL IN THE BLANKS

Fill in the blanks in each statement using the words in the box below.
Not all of them are required and some may be used more than once, so choose carefully.

risk assessment	gowns
body fluids	hand hygiene
disposable	replaced
following	masks
removed	start
single-use	reusable
soiled	care plan
preventable	management
portable	contaminated
point	unnecessary
line	policy
floor	sharp-
table	inevitable
necessary	

23 Personal protective equipment is _____,_____ clothing and equipment; it includes _____, gloves, aprons, goggles, visors and _____.

24 When considering infection control, a _____ is required to determine which PPE is most appropriate for the task/situation, depending on what the wearer might be exposed to, e.g. blood/ _____.

25 The choice of PPE should be put on at the _____ of the procedure and removed promptly at the end of the procedure.

26 If it becomes torn, damaged or _____ during the procedure, it should be _____ ; _____ should always be carried out prior to and _____ removal of P P E.

27 A sharps injury is any incident in which a healthcare worker is stuck by a needle or other sharp instrument which penetrates the skin and which is _____ with potentially infected blood. All sharps injuries are considered to be potentially _____.

28 Provision of _____ sharps containers for all staff at all times is crucial to allow used sharps to be disposed of at the _____ of use. These must not be filled above the _____ indicating that they are full. Containers in public areas must not be placed on the _____ and should be located in a safe position.

29 Underreporting is a serious threat to _____ of such injuries; prompt reporting according to local _____ is essential.

30 Eliminate the _____ use of sharps by implementing changes in practice and providing, where practicable _____ free devices or safer needle technologies which retract or shield needles after use.

ANSWERS

TRUE OR FALSE?

1   **Bacteria grow faster under gloved than ungloved hands.** ✔

The hands of someone wearing gloves are well suited to bacterial growth, being warm and moist. Hands should be cleaned before and after every care activity, and after any activity that may result in them becoming contaminated (i.e. after exposure to body fluids), regardless of whether gloves are used. Gloves used in health care may have holes in them, allowing infectious agents to pass between the carer's hands and the patient, in either direction.

2   **Surgical site infections contribute to nosocomial infections.** ✔

A nosocomial infection is any infection that is a result of treatment in a hospital or a healthcare service unit. Infections are considered nosocomial if they first appear 48 hours or more after hospital admission or within 30 days after discharge. This type of infection is also known as a healthcare-associated infection (HCAI). For this reason, it is important not to disturb the dressing for the first 48 hours on surgical wounds healing by primary intention.

3   **When washing hands, using a nailbrush helps to remove bacteria and leaves hands cleaner.** ✖

Nailbrushes must not be used for routine hand washing. Continuous use of nailbrushes damages the skin, which will then harbour bacteria. Nailbrushes also become contaminated and therefore act as a source of cross-infection. If used in specific circumstances, such as prior to surgery, they must be single-use and sterile.

4   **Gloves may be washed and reused for the same patient.** ✖

Gloves should not be washed or re-used, and must be discarded following the correct local policy.

5   **Alcohol-based rubs are very useful when working with a patient who has *Clostridium difficile* infection.** ✖

Alcohol-based rubs are not reliable against any spore-forming bacteria such as *Clostridium difficile*. For this reason, they are not recommended for use with patients suspected of having *Clostridium difficile* infection or any patient with diarrhoea while awaiting confirmation of infection.

6 | **Artificial nails are acceptable if kept clean.** ✖

Nail varnish and artificial nails harbour microbes that cannot be effectively removed and must not be worn.

7 | **Hands should be wetted under running water and liquid soap applied before rubbing together vigorously.**

Hands should be moistened in advance of applying the soap to aid foaming. Liquid soap must be in a closed container so that it does not come into contact with the user's hands; bars of soap are easily contaminated and should not be used. Fingertips, inter-digital spaces, and thumbs have been identified as the most frequently missed areas when performing hand hygiene. Pointing hands downwards is important to prevent contaminated water running back up the arms.

8 | **If disposable towels are unavailable, it is acceptable to use the patient's towel to dry your hands.** ✖

Hands must be effectively dried, as wet hands provide the ideal environment for bacterial growth. The choice of towel is also important; it should be disposable, as communal towels may harbour bacteria. When disposing of a paper towel, take care not to re-contaminate your hands from sources such as the bin, paper towel holder or taps. Under no circumstances should the patient's towel be used.

9 | **The complete process of hand washing should take no less than 40 seconds.**

Hand washing to ensure thorough cleanliness should take between 40 and 60 seconds; the process of using an alcohol-based rub should take between 20 and 30 seconds.

10 | **The non-touch technique can be incorporated as part of a clean procedure.** ✔

The non-touch technique can be incorporated as part of a clean procedure, i.e. the ends of sterile connections or other items that could contaminate a sterile field should not be touched.

11 | **When using sterile gloves, hand washing is not crucial.** ✖

The National Patient Safety Agency (2008) stresses the importance of hand hygiene at all times regardless of whether gloves are being used.

MULTIPLE CHOICE
Correct answers identified in bold italics

12 **The most common way of spreading infection in a healthcare environment is via:**

a) overuse of antibiotics   b) patient isolation

c) hands of healthcare staff   d) toilet seats

The importance of hand hygiene has been repeatedly emphasized, including by the World Health Organization (WHO). The point of care has been identified as the crucial aspect, as this represents the time when the risk of cross-infection is greatest; the point of care refers to the patient's immediate environment (zones). The WHO highlights five crucial moments when hands should be cleaned: before patient contact, before an aseptic task, after exposure risk to body fluids, after patient contact, and after contact with patient surroundings.

13 **The choice of personal protective equipment is made by:**

a) the nurse after assessing the situation

b) the doctor in charge of the patient

c) the infection control team

d) the ward manager

The choice of personal protective equipment is made after a risk assessment has been carried out. The nurse will then use the risk assessment to identify the correct protocol that has been drawn up by the infection control team for that specific area. The importance of adhering to local protocols is important, as these protocols and policies are drawn up based on recent evidence to ensure the best response to any situation by the identified infection control team.

14 **Isolation nursing is:**

a) intended to prevent the spread of infection to patients and others

b) wearing personal protective clothing at all times

c) wearing gloves and aprons during all patient contact

d) ensuring no visitors are allowed

Isolation nursing is a term used to describe the separation of patients with an infection from others to prevent the spread of the condition. It is also used to reduce the risk of transmission of infections from others to the immune-compromised patient. Patients are usually isolated in separate rooms; if this is not possible, they are grouped together and this is termed 'bed isolation'. The specific local protocols need to be referred to when identifying the need for isolation nursing.

15 **Gloves should be worn:**

a) *for handling items contaminated with blood*
b) when feeding a patient with MRSA
c) when administering oral medications
d) when charting the observations of a patient in isolation

Gloves should be worn when touching blood and bodily fluids and when handling items contaminated with these. Gloves must be changed after contact with each client and hands washed immediately; the use of gloves does not reduce the need for hand washing.

16 **Sterile gloves should be used when:**

a) carrying out urinary catheter care
b) *inserting a urinary catheter*
c) erecting intravenous fluids
d) performing venepuncture

Sterile gloves should be employed for all procedures where asepsis is needed, e.g. during urinary catheter insertion or in theatre. When the gloves are required as a protective measure because the procedure involves the risk of contamination with blood or bodily fluids, such as urinary catheter care or venepuncture, non-sterile gloves are adequate and more cost-effective.

17 **Which of the following contributes to the prevention of oro-faecal contamination?**

a) drinking only bottled water
b) disposable rubbish bags
c) *provision of hot water, soap, and towels*
d) non-sterile gloves

Poor hand hygiene after toileting is a contributing factor to oro-faecal contamination; lack of facilities has been found to be a major contributing factor. The provision of soap and hot water with disposable towels – rather than a non-disposable towel, which may harbour bacteria – is essential for reducing the risk of this type of contamination.

18 **'Superbugs' are:**

a) any infection acquired in the healthcare environment
b) *pathogens that have become resistant to treatment*
c) cockroaches found in healthcare environments
d) specific viral infections

'Superbugs' are not new bacteria but bacteria that have developed and gained a resistance to the various common treatments, making them more difficult to eradicate. The key point about many 'superbugs' is that they are not generally more aggressive, simply that they are more resistant to treatment. These pathogens are present both in the healthcare environment and the wider community.

19 **MRSA stands for:**

a) microorganisms resistant to specific antibiotics
b) methicillin-resistant Staphylococcus aureus
c) micro-resistant *Staphylococcus aureus*
d) methicillin-reactive *Staphylococcus aureus*

MRSA is any strain of *Staphylococcus aureus* that has developed a resistance to certain antibiotics, including the penicillins (methicillin, dicloxacillin, nafcillin, oxacillin, etc.) and the cephalosporins. MRSA is especially troublesome in hospitals and nursing homes where patients with open wounds, invasive devices, and weakened immune systems are at greater risk of infection than the general public.

20 **A care bundle is:**

a) a checklist
b) a small, essential set of evidence-based practices
c) a parcel of local policies
d) a set of patient care procedures

The concept of 'bundles' was developed by the Institute for Healthcare Improvement (IHI). When performed collectively, care bundles have been shown to improve patient outcomes, and for this reason a care bundle is small, specific, and evidence-based; this enables the healthcare provider to be more reliable in the delivery of care. The use of care bundles is particularly important when patients are undergoing treatments that pose a high risk of infection. Bundles are not checklists and vice versa; they must only be changed or added to following strict criteria and agreement.

21 **The aseptic non-touch technique involves the use of:**

a) face masks　*b) sterile gloves*　c) dressing pack
d) sodium chloride

Aseptic non-touch technique (ANTT) is designed to prevent the entry of pathogenic organisms into susceptible sites. When carrying out ANTT, the nurse should plan ahead to prepare self, equipment, environment, and patient to reduce any unnecessary interruptions throughout the procedure. ANTT may be achieved using sterile products but does not always involve the use of a dressing pack.

22 An aseptic technique should be carried out for procedures such as:

a) *surgical wound dressing*
b) urinary catheter care
c) blood glucose monitoring
d) administration of eye drops

For all procedures where asepsis is required, sterile gloves need to be used; where the risk is from contamination with blood or body fluids, non-sterile gloves can be used.

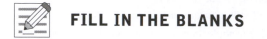

FILL IN THE BLANKS

23 Personal protective equipment (PPE) is *disposable, single-use* clothing and equipment; it includes *gowns*, gloves, aprons, goggles, visors and *masks*.

24 When considering infection control, a *risk assessment* is required to determine which PPE is most appropriate for the task/situation, depending on what the wearer might be exposed to, e.g. blood/*body fluids*.

25 The choice of PPE should be put on at the *start* of the procedure and removed promptly at the end of the procedure.

26 If it becomes torn, damaged or *soiled* during the procedure, it should be *replaced; hand hygiene* should always be carried out prior to and *following* removal of PPE.

It is important to select the most appropriate PPE for the procedure according to local policy so that adequate protection is provided without being wasteful. All PPE must be disposed of on removal according to local policy.

27 A sharps injury is any incident in which a healthcare worker is stuck by a needle or other sharp instrument which penetrates the skin and which is *contaminated* with potentially infected blood. All sharps injuries are considered to be potentially *preventable.*

28 Provision of *portable* sharps containers for all staff at all times is crucial to allow used sharps to be disposed of at the *point* of use. These must not be filled above the *line* indicating that they are full. Containers in public areas must not be placed on the *floor* and should be located in a safe position.

29 Underreporting is a serious threat to *management* of such injuries; prompt reporting according to local *policy* is essential.

30 Eliminate the *unnecessary* use of sharps by implementing changes in practice and providing, where practicable, *sharp*-free devices or safer needle technologies which retract or shield needles after use.

The risk of sharps injuries can be greatly reduced when local policies are adhered to. Recommendations include not passing sharps from one person to another, and not bending, breaking, dismantling or re-sheathing needles. Sharps must be disposed of at the point of use and the containers stored safely away from public areas. Unnecessary use of sharps should be avoided through the use of safety devices such as vacuum blood collection systems.

2 Risk assessment – moving and handling

INTRODUCTION

Many nurses regularly experience back pain and many manual handling incidents cause nurses to take long periods of time off work because of injuries sustained. It is clear, therefore, that moving and handling patients can present a threat to the health and well-being of nurses. As is considered good practice elsewhere, these risks must be assessed, managed and minimized or, ideally, eliminated.

The dilemma for nurses is that failure to move a patient may have negative consequences for the patient, but moving the patient is potentially dangerous for the nurse. It is clear that the rates of back, neck and joint injury (including wrist, knee and ankle) among healthcare staff are high, with inevitable consequences for those staff and the health service as a whole. A period of 'safe' lifting techniques was tried by decision makers in an attempt to reduce the injury rate and associated absenteeism; however, it became apparent that the rate of injury did not fall significantly when adopting these 'safe' techniques. There was a paradigm shift, in that it became clear that lifting a patient could never be safe, so other techniques and devices were developed to make this necessary aspect of patient care safer. It is important, therefore, for nurses to have a clear understanding of what the law and good practice guidelines demand of nurses as employees, as well as of their employers, in relation to safe moving and handling practices.

Useful resources

National Back Exchange (NBE):
http://www.nationalbackexchange.org.uk

Health & Safety Executive Short guide to regulations and risk assessment:
http://www.hse.gov.uk/pubns/indg143.pdf

Health & Safety Executive Manual handling assessment charts:
http://www.hse.gov.uk/pubns/indg383.pdf

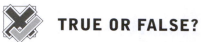

TRUE OR FALSE?

Are the following statements true or false?

1   Back pain is the only type of injury suffered by nurses in moving and handling patients.

2   Ergonomics is the study of how to lift patients safely.

3   Moving and handling patients is inherently unsafe and should be avoided at all costs.

4   Completion of a risk assessment form guarantees that all risk factors have been adequately identified.

5   Refusal to lift a patient would be deemed 'professional misconduct'.

6   Moving and handling risk assessment is not just 'good practice' but has potentially serious legal ramifications for all concerned in handling operations (nurse, employer and patient).

7   The Manual Handling Operations Regulations (MHOR) 1992 (Amended 2004) relate only to the movement of inanimate objects.

8 Pushing or pulling is not considered to be a handling operation so, for example, moving a bed or chair need not form part of a risk assessment.

9 Risk assessment is an intuitive process and, therefore, requires no special knowledge, skill or training.

10 Risk refers to the degree to which negative events *only* are likely to occur.

a b c d MULTIPLE CHOICE

Identify one correct answer for each of the following.

11 As part of risk assessment, an employer is required *only* to:

a) reduce risk, since its complete avoidance is not possible

b) avoid risk entirely for employees

c) avoid risk when possible, but otherwise reduce it

d) avoid the need for the task if possible, assess the degree of risk and reduce it to the lowest practicable level, then keep it under constant review

12 Which of the following movements of the spine is most dangerous for the nurse? A movement that requires:

a) bending and twisting

b) pulling and pushing

c) stooping

d) reaching upwards

13 The act of assisting patients from sitting to standing:

a) presents little risk to staff

b) presents little risk to patients

c) poses an increased risk of injury to staff

d) is relatively low and therefore requires little special knowledge or training

14 According to the MHOR (1992) (Amended 2004), a risk assessment should identify:

a) tasks to be carried out, who will carry them out and how the patient will be moved and handled

b) only how the patient will be moved and handled

c) who will move and handle the patient

d) the types of operation required to meet the patient's needs

15 Moving and handling risk assessment is best carried out by:

a) any nurse involved in care

b) a physiotherapist

c) any competent member of staff who is familiar with the operations in question

d) the nurse in charge

16 Generally, moving and handling risk assessment is best recorded, but the assessment need not necessarily be recorded if:

a) the department is busy

b) the proposed operation is of low risk, will last only a short time, and would require a disproportionate length of time to record

c) the staff involved agree

d) it does not involve handling a patient

17 A moving and handling risk assessment is normally reviewed if:

a) the patient is transferred to another department

b) there is reason to believe it is no longer valid

c) 30 days have elapsed since it was first carried out

d) 14 days have elapsed since it was first carried out

18 If a valid risk assessment carried out by a competent person reveals that a hoist should be used to move a patient, a competent nurse may decide not to use the hoist if:

a) three members of staff are available to execute the move

b) the hoist is currently unavailable and the patient wants/needs to be moved immediately

c) ordered not to by a senior nurse

d) the nurse **must** use the hoist

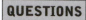

FILL IN THE BLANKS

Fill in the blanks in each statement using the words in the box below.
Not all of them are required and some may be used more than once, so choose carefully.

rest	training
space	bulky
posture	pregnant
strength	bending
shift	floor
lowering	lighting

When carrying out a moving and handling risk assessment, the following are *some* of the questions a nurse should try to answer in relation to the task, the load, the environment and the individual capabilities of the people to carry out the moving and handling operation.

19 Does the task involve unsatisfactory body _____ , such as bending or twisting?

20 Does the task involve excessive lifting or _____ distances?

21 Does the task involve inadequate _____ periods?

22 Is the load _____ or difficult to grasp?

23 Is the load likely to _____ suddenly?

24 Are the _____ constraints preventing good posture?

25 Are there poor _____ conditions?

26 Do individuals require _____ to do this work?

27 Might it put those who are _____ at risk?

28 Does the individual require special _____ ?

ANSWERS

TRUE OR FALSE?

1 | **Back pain is the only type of injury suffered by nurses in moving and handling patients.**

According to the Health and Safety Executive (HSE), sprains/strains account for 69% of work-acquired moving and handling injuries that result in more than 3 days' absence from work. However, injuries to fingers, arms, shoulders, hands, knees, ankles, feet and neck, together account for a higher proportion of injuries. Therefore, risk assessment should take account of possible injury when operating hoists, connecting slings, moving beds and bedsides, using wheelchairs, etc. It is also important for any risk assessment to acknowledge that these injuries can occur to patients as well as staff.

2 | **Ergonomics is the study of how to lift patients safely.**

The work patterns in many departments demand that 'tasks' be accomplished by certain (unwritten) times. This can have an effect on how nurses practise and organize workloads. Ergonomics recognizes that it is inadequate simply to examine tasks to be done or numbers of people to accomplish the tasks. It recognizes that people have differing capabilities and potential; they work in an environment that can affect them and their relationships. Sometimes, it is better to make a change in the environment for a change to occur in people. Therefore, any moving and handling risk assessment must use an ergonomic model, and take account of the environment within which people work, in order to maintain health and safety.

3 | **Moving and handling patients is inherently unsafe and should be avoided at all costs.**

Moving and handling patients carries with it the risk that nurses or the patient may suffer an acute injury or, more likely, injury that results from the cumulative effect of repeatedly carrying out the same operation over weeks, months or even years. This means that an activity may not, at first, appear risky and the danger may become apparent only with hindsight, which, of course, is too late. The effect of these injuries can vary from minor to long term, even career-threatening. Legislation such as the Health and Safety at Work Act 1974, Management of Health and Safety at Work Regulations 1999, and Manual Handling Operations Regulations 1992 (Updated 2004), together with various other statutes and conventions is recognition of the fact that people can get injured in the course of their work. How to respond to that is more complex, however, but avoiding it at all costs is not possible. Therefore, while nurses must not compromise their own health and safety, they must be ready to assess the risk and act accordingly.

4 | **Completion of a risk assessment form guarantees that all risk factors have been adequately identified.** ✖

Completing risk assessment can give structure, procedure and routine to a potentially hazardous activity and it helps nurses think clearly about how to move and handle patients safely. The risk assessment should be committed to paper but the paper record must not become the point of the exercise. A fully completed 'form' that is not consulted or modified again is of no real value. Continuously thinking about risk management and reduction means that, as risks emerge or recede, a nurse is more likely to be vigilant to changing situations and risks will be identified. It is 'thinking' on the part of the nurse that brings this about, not just writing.

5 | **Refusal to lift a patient would be deemed 'professional misconduct'.** ✖

Nurses must practise at all times in accordance with the NMC Code of Conduct (NMC 2008). They are also required, as employees, to take care of their own well-being and that of colleagues (Health and Safety at Work Act 1974). This can sometimes present a dilemma, whereby a nurse may feel obliged to do everything possible for a patient, even at risk to one's own health; clearly, nurses should not do this. There is precedent in professional conduct committee hearings in which nurses, having refused to execute what they believed to be a dangerous manoeuvre, were found not guilty of professional misconduct. However, any nurse embarking on such a course must be able to show how this decision was arrived at. This can be achieved only after a thorough risk assessment that identifies all the areas considered.

6 | **Moving and handling risk assessment is not just 'good practice' but has potentially serious legal ramifications for all concerned in handling operations (nurse, employer and the patient).**

Having acknowledged that moving and handling can result in a range of injuries to nurses and, potentially, to patients, it is to be acknowledged also that injured people sometimes seek redress in law for the injuries they have sustained. There is also a clear financial cost. Therefore, all concerned must assess and reduce the risks identified. A nurse who engages in complex moving and handling operations without being able to show evidence of prior risk assessment may be breaking the law, is certainly not adhering to accepted standards of practice in this area and, in this instance, may be guilty of professional misconduct. They may also be compromising any legal action they may feel entitled to take afterwards, or at least have possible awards reduced because of 'contributory negligence' – that is, the degree to which a court may decide that a nurse was responsible for causing their own injury.

7 | The Manual Handling Operations Regulations (MHOR) 1992 (Amended 2004) relate only to the movement of inanimate objects.

The MHOR provide the basis for a thorough and wide-ranging risk assessment of moving and handling activities. It is clear that they relate to all forms of moving and handling to be carried out by workers in all spheres of work and industry. Some believe they are mostly to do with handling inanimate loads. However, it is clear that they relate to any activity in which a person has to support all or most of the weight of a discrete moveable object. The regulations set out clearly that a load may be inanimate (a box) or animate, a patient receiving medical attention, and that risks can be found in all workplaces, including care homes.

8 | Pushing or pulling is not considered to be a handling operation so, for example, moving a bed or chair need not form part of a risk assessment.

The MHOR set out that the regulations apply to all manual handling activities including lifting, lowering, pushing, pulling, carrying and moving. Therefore, moving a heavy patient in a bed or wheelchair may contain an element of risk to the handler. While a hoist must *never* be used to transport a patient over distance, pulling and pushing it around a bed area may contain some element of risk. Also, moving furniture and equipment around can be considered a potential cause of injury, especially for those who work in departments where this happens many times as part of the daily routine, e.g. wheeling beds in and out of theatre and recovery areas, or short stay areas where patient transfer is a frequent occurrence.

9 | Risk assessment is an intuitive process and, therefore, requires no special knowledge, skill or training.

The MHOR set out that risk assessment should be done between employers and employees, and refer to the 'need to use their experience of the work being done'. The work involved in a healthcare setting is specialist and requires specialist knowledge, skill and training. Therefore, only people with special skills and knowledge of the area can assess the particular risks involved and how they can be reduced or managed. The regulations make clear that staff should be properly trained in meeting the mobility needs of patients with whom they are working and, by extension, they should be trained in assessing the risk associated with moving or handling those patients. A nurse carrying out a risk assessment in a spinal injury would clearly need awareness of different potential risks and solutions than a nurse working in a day procedure unit. Therefore, Nursing Students need to learn about moving and handling risk assessment from differing perspectives while on different placements.

10 **Risk refers to the degree to which negative events *only* are likely to occur.** ✓

When one thinks of risk, one usually considers the possibility that something negative might happen. Therefore, risk assessment is a structured attempt to identify risks or dangers inherent in a situation, quantify the likelihood that this may happen, and decide if the activity producing the risk can be avoided; if it cannot be avoided, then one is obliged to reduce the risk, and therefore, the likelihood of a bad outcome (e.g. someone becoming injured). To help achieve this, a risk assessment should identify the necessary actions needed to reduce the risk, who will carry out these actions, specifically how the patient will be moved or handled and, ideally, the extent to which the patient may help with the move, as well as the specific handling equipment to be used (MHOR 1992).

MULTIPLE CHOICE

Correct answers identified in bold italics

11 **As part of risk assessment, an employer is required *only* to:**

a) reduce risk, since its complete avoidance is not possible

b) avoid risk entirely for employees

c) avoid risk when possible, but otherwise reduce it

d) ***avoid the need for the task if possible, assess the degree of risk and reduce it to the lowest practicable level, then keep it under constant review***

The Manual Handling Operations Regulations (MHOR) 1992 (Amended 2004) require an employer to make suitable risk assessment of the possible risks to the health and safety of their employees, associated with moving and handling; if this risk assessment reveals handling-related risks, employers are obliged to comply with the regulations. This means the elimination of the need for the task to be carried out, where possible. If the handling operation cannot be avoided, a detailed assessment must be carried out to reduce the risk as far as is reasonably practicable. In a healthcare setting, it is likely that most moving and handling cannot be avoided but nurses should be alert to the possibility that some things could be done in a different way; perhaps a patient may be able to assist more than initially realized, thus reducing the risk of injury. The regulations also make clear that risk assessments need to be recorded and the record made readily accessible and kept under review.

12　**Which of the following movements of the spine is most dangerous for the nurse? A movement that requires:**

a) bending and twisting　　b) pulling and pushing　　c) stooping

d) reaching upwards

Generally, the most common movements involve flexion (bending forward) or extension (stretching the shoulders back, slightly behind the hips). There is also the possibility of rotation, whereby the shoulders are directed in a different direction to the hips (twisting). Any or all of these movements can be risky, especially when carried out under load. However, a nurse should consider that, if bending forward and simultaneously twisting the spine is necessary to carry out a handling manoeuvre, then this is especially dangerous and should be assessed again to find another way to carry out the move. This type of movement may be forced on a nurse when working in confined spaces such as a bathroom or toilet cubicle or where a patient has fallen. In such circumstances, pausing to think of a way to move a patient or clearing the environment first may help avoid injury.

13　**The act of assisting patients from sitting to standing:**

a)　presents little risk to staff

b)　presents little risk to patients

c)　poses an increased risk of injury to staff

d)　is relatively low and therefore requires little special knowledge or training

Sometimes a handling operation can seem relatively innocuous and straightforward, resulting in it being underestimated as a risky manoeuvre. There are many situations in which a patient may need some assistance in getting from a sitting to a standing position, and, since this is a handling operation, under the terms of the MHOR it should be assessed for any risk it may pose. There is evidence that providing care and assistance to those who cannot rise from sitting to standing unaided presents an increased risk of injury to the carers involved. When this manoeuvre is required, it is recommended that two handlers be involved, since one handler aiding a patient who cannot offer much help poses extra danger.

14　**According to the MHOR (1992) (Amended 2004), a risk assessment should identify:**

a)　tasks to be carried out, who will carry them out and how the patient will be moved and handled

b)　only how the patient will be moved and handled

c)　who will move and handle the patient

d)　the types of operation required to meet the patient's needs

Under the terms of MHOR, assessments should contain information about: the task to be accomplished; the load (patient) to be handled or moved; the environment in which the activity will take place; the individual capacity of the people involved; and any other relevant factors, such as the need for special precautions (e.g. use of personal protective equipment). The conclusion of the risk assessment should detail how many staff will be required for the various handling operations, whether or not the patient can assist, perhaps patient preferences and what specific handling equipment should be used.

15 Moving and handling risk assessment is best carried out by:

a) any nurse involved in care

b) a physiotherapist

c) any competent member of staff who is familiar with the operations in question

d) the nurse in charge

Moving and handling risk assessment must be carried out by employers to identify the precise nature of the work involved and what is required of their employees. Risk assessment will require knowledge of the legal requirements and the specific demands of the MHOR. Therefore, such an assessment may need to be carried out by a manager with special training, or a specially trained health and safety advisor or ergonomist. An assessor will also need to identify high-risk activities and suggest practical steps to reduce those risks. Competent, experienced nurses who are familiar with the daily demands of their department can perform such an assessment for patients when necessary.

16 Generally, moving and handling risk assessment is best recorded, but the assessment need not necessarily be recorded if:

a) the department is busy

b) the proposed operation is of low risk, will last only a short time, and would require a disproportionate length of time to record (MHOR 1992)

c) the staff involved agree

d) it does not involve handling a patient

Many caring activities are recurring and can be foreseen but some may not be. This may mean that some handling episodes are required that were not planned for, such as when a patient falls or an emergency situation develops. It would clearly be difficult, and perhaps counterproductive, to begin recording a risk assessment when more immediate action is required. Similarly, if every small patient encounter was to be subjected to risk assessment, the time used would be disproportionate to the benefit, and records would become unnecessarily bulky and perhaps unhelpful. These decisions are best taken at the time by experienced, competent staff.

17 **A moving and handling risk assessment is normally reviewed if:**

a) the patient is transferred to another department
b) *there is reason to believe it is no longer valid*
c) 30 days have elapsed since it was first carried out
d) 14 days have elapsed since it was first carried out

Risk assessments must be kept up to date and be reviewed if there is a change in a patient's condition or capabilities. The regulations make clear that a review is necessary if an injury occurs due to a handling operation. They also make clear that a review is necessary if a change in the condition of a member of staff may make them more vulnerable to injury, such as the development of a medical condition or becoming pregnant. There is no set time frame for reviews to be conducted.

18 **If a valid risk assessment carried out by a competent person reveals that a hoist should be used to move a patient, a competent nurse may decide not to use the hoist if:**

a) three members of staff are available to execute the move
b) the hoist is currently unavailable and the patient wants/needs to be moved immediately
c) ordered not to by a senior nurse
d) *the nurse must use the hoist*

As employees, nurses have duties under the Health and Safety at Work Act 1974, the MHOR 1992 (Amended 2004) and Management of Health and Safety at Work Regulations 1999; they are obliged to make full and proper use of any system of work provided by an employer; they must also take reasonable care for their own health and that of others who may be affected by their activities. Nurses must also cooperate with employers to enable them to meet their obligations in relation to health and safety. Nurses are also obliged to make use of appropriate equipment provided for them by their employer.

FILL IN THE BLANKS

19 **Does the task involve unsatisfactory body *posture*, such as bending or twisting?**

Any operation that causes a nurse to have to engage in excessive bending or twisting, particularly under load, increases the risk of back injury. Even short manoeuvres, if they have to be repeated many times in a day, can have a cumulative damaging effect on a nurse's back.

20 **Does the task involve excessive lifting or *lowering* distances?**

A weight to be moved will require greater force to be exerted by the handler if it is a lot lower, higher or far away from the lumbar spine. Therefore, moving a weight from the floor, such as helping a fallen patient, assisting a patient from a bath, lifting a box containing equipment, can be potentially damaging to the nurse. Similarly, continually having to place objects onto, or retrieve objects from, high shelves should also be considered high-risk activities and special arrangements should be made, including the use of special equipment (e.g. hoists) or rearranging the environment so as to avoid the need for lifting (bales of heavy bed linen?) onto or from high shelves.

21 **Does the task involve inadequate *rest* periods?**

The organization of work may allow insufficient rest or recovery periods for the carers involved, particularly if they are working in a small team of two. If this is an established system of work that is repeated on many days each week, the cumulative effect on the back can be damaging. Using equipment supplied by employers, attempting to be more flexible in organizing work patterns, and teaching simple exercises to staff that can be performed easily can help moderate some of these risks.

22 **Is the load *bulky* or difficult to grasp?**

Sometimes the weight of a load to be moved is less crucial than the fact that its characteristics may make it awkward to grasp. Consider moving a patient who is not particularly heavy, but has very painful joints due to arthritis; the compromises made in handling such a person so as to avoid exacerbating their pain may cause a nurse to overlook usual moving and handling 'rules'. Similarly, the human form is not designed for easy moving and handling and has a range of shapes and sizes. A risk assessment should take account of the particular issues that may need to be dealt with in handling a patient, including their weight, height, mental state, ability/willingness to cooperate, their medical condition and whether or not they want to be moved.

23 **Is the load likely to *shift* suddenly?**

Patients who know what nurses are doing when attempting to move them are often able to cooperate. However, a patient may become frightened and suddenly begin to resist during the handling operation. The patient's condition may suddenly change, for instance, they may begin to fall to the floor or, when being helped from bed, may suddenly faint. A competent, experienced nurse can help avoid this risk by conducting a thorough prior moving and handling risk assessment.

24 **Are the *space* constraints preventing good posture?**

A possible feature of moving and handling accidents is lack of space. This may be because nurses have to work in an environment not specifically designed for a moving and handling activity, such as the patient's home.

Occasionally, a patient may fall or become incapacitated in an enclosed space (a toilet cubicle) and this will present difficulties for staff because risky body postures may be adopted (bending and twisting). Nurses should recognize space constraints as a possible threat to their health and safety when carrying out a risk assessment.

25 Are there poor *lighting* conditions?

Nurses work mostly in well-lit environments. However, in some cases, environmental lighting may not be ideal. This may be the case when working in a patient's own home or when on night duty with a failed night-light. Nurses should be aware that, when working in low or inadequate lighting conditions, accidents may happen and care should be taken in assuming that a patient's vision in low-light conditions is adequate to enable full cooperation.

26 Do individuals require *training* to do this work?

Moving and handling patients is specialist work and carries with it potential risk. This means that such work also requires specialist knowledge, skill and information, and the MHOR 1992 (amended 2004) recognize this fact. Nurses should be sure they have had adequate training and education before undertaking any of these activities, and they should also be sure their knowledge of the relevant legislation and standards is sufficient to enable compliance with the very highest standards of moving and handling practice.

27 Might it put those who are *pregnant* at risk?

As part of any moving and handling risk assessment, managers and staff should recognize that the stresses associated with moving patients may place those who are pregnant at special risk. Any training regimes should make all staff aware of their responsibilities to their own health and that of their unborn baby; staff should feel freely able to make this fact known at a time of their choosing and colleagues should also take this into consideration.

28 Does the individual require special *strength*?

Some nurses believe there is merit in the routine deployment of natural strength and vigour as the solution to a moving and handling problem. The MHOR accept that well-intentioned modifications in an emergency may be acceptable; however, the routine application of physical strength in moving and handling situations is neither good nor intelligent practice. Except in an emergency situation, the usual rules of risk assessment, and adherence to legislation and standards of practice, are always to be expected.

3 | Administration of medicines

INTRODUCTION

The administration of medications is one of the interventions that the nurse does to improve a patient's health. The administration of medications can also be associated with error and it is therefore important that nurses have the knowledge associated with the correct administration of drugs and medications. The Nursing and Midwifery Council (NMC) have set standards for safe practice in the management and administration of medicines by registered nurses, midwives and specialist community public health nurses. It is important that you, as a nursing student, are aware of these standards, as failure to adhere to the NMC standards will almost certainly affect your patients and may put your potential registration at risk.

This chapter does not deal with drug calculations, as other publications deal specifically with this topic. Rather, this chapter seeks to test you on the important legislative and professional aspects of drug administration and to help you to minimize medication-related risk.

Useful resources

Standards for medicines management:
http://www.nmc-uk.org/Publications/Standards/

Nurses! Test Yourself in Essential Calculation Skills

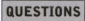 **TRUE OR FALSE?**

Are the following statements true or false?

 1   The National Patient Safety Agency (NPSA) monitors and advises on issues connected with the administration of medicines.

 2   The NMC issues guidance on the administration of medicines to doctors and nurses.

 3   When administering a drug, a registered nurse is personally accountable for his or her actions.

 4   Nurses need a working understanding of medicines administered, therapeutic dosages and side-effects.

 5   Medicines administered by a nursing student must be under the direct supervision of a doctor.

 6   When in use, the medicine trolley must not be left unattended.

 7   The pharmacist has the right to audit the medicine cupboard at any time.

 8   A nurse cannot refuse to administer a medicine when the prescription is signed by a doctor.

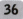

9 The police will be contacted if there is any suspicion of drug irregularity in any clinical setting.

10 Most adverse incidents in hospital are due to drug irregularities.

![ab/cd] MULTIPLE CHOICE

Identify one correct answer for each of the following.

11 If a patient has an allergy, the NPSA states this should be:

   a) written on the identity armband only

   b) written on the identity armband and verbally reported to colleagues

   c) written on the identity armband and on the medicine kardex

   d) written on the identity armband, in the patient case notes and the medicine chart

12 As a nursing student, when checking the patient's identity against the medicine kardex (medication administration record), you should:

   a) bring the kardex with you to the patient and check as per NPSA guidelines

   b) leave the kardex with the registered nurse and then verbally check the patient's identity as per NPSA guidelines

   c) ask the patient to identify themselves and then administer the drug

   d) leave the kardex with the registered nurse and then verbally check the patient's identity and wait for the registered nurse to confirm

13 If a patient is nil by mouth:

   a) all drugs should be withheld

   b) all oral drugs should be withheld

   c) the decision to withhold oral drugs should be taken in conjunction with the doctor

   d) if drugs are prescribed, they should be given regardless

14 If a patient has a temporary tracheotomy and is on regular nebulizers, these should be:

a) withheld until the tracheotomy is reversed

b) given via a regular oxygen mask over mouth and nose

c) given via a tracheotomy mask

d) given via a non-rebreathing mask over the tracheotomy

15 As a nursing student, when administering a drug, it is:

a) never acceptable not to know specific drugs that you are administering

b) acceptable not to know specific drugs that you are administering as long as the registered nurse knows the drug

c) acceptable not to know the drug you are administering as long as the patient knows the drug

d) acceptable not to know the drug you are administering as long as the carer/relative knows the drug

16 If a patient has difficulty swallowing:

a) all drugs should be withheld

b) alternate routes should be considered

c) tablets should be crushed

d) the patient should be persuaded to take a large volume of water to help to swallow medication

17 If a patient brings his or her own medications into hospital, the medications:

a) should be taken from the patient and sent to the hospital pharmacy for disposal

b) should be put in the medicine trolley and treated as ward stock

c) should be taken from the patient and sent to the hospital pharmacy for storage

d) are the property of the patient to whom they were supplied and must not be taken without consent

18 The deltoid muscle should be used when:

a) a slow uptake of the medication is required

b) a fast uptake of the medication is required

c) 4–5 millilitres of medication are to be given

d) 10 millilitres of medication are to be given

19 Needles are colour-coded according to their gauge. When administrating an intramuscular injection, it is generally acceptable to use:

a) a blue needle

b) an orange needle

c) a grey needle

d) a green needle

FILL IN THE BLANKS

Fill in the blanks in each statement using the words in the box below.
Not all of them are required, so choose carefully.

skin	fat
dermis	skeletal muscle
smooth muscle	slowly
rapidly	bloodstream
epidural	subcutaneous
intercostal	albumin
haemoglobin	hypoalbuminaemia
hyperalbuminaemia	metabolism
digestion	children
older adult	liver
stomach	renal
cardiac	endocrine

20 A subcutaneous (SC) injection means a drug Is given beneath the
_____ into the connective issue or _____ immediately underlying the
_____.

21 Intramuscular (IM) administration means a drug is injected into
_____. Absorption occurs more _____ than with SC injection
because of greater tissue blood flow.

22 The intravenous route is an injection directly into the _____ and
produces an immediate response.

23 Epidural administration of a drug means that it is injected via a small catheter into the _____ space.

24 As a drug enters the bloodstream, it binds to protein, mainly _____.

25 The factors influencing drug-protein binding are the degree of drug binding, the competition for binding sites and _____.

26 The process of chemically inactivating a drug by converting it into a more water-soluble compound or metabolite is known as _____.

27 _____ with immature metabolizing systems and the _____ with degenerative enzyme function experience depressed metabolism.

28 The _____ is a major metabolizing organ for drugs.

29 Abnormal clearance of a drug may be anticipated when a client has _____ function impairment.

ANSWERS

TRUE OR FALSE?

1 | **The National Patient Safety Agency (NPSA) monitors and advises on issues connected to the administration of medicines.** ✓

NPSA aims to improve patient safety by informing, supporting and influencing organizations and people working in the health sector. NPSA is linked to the Department of Health and covers the United Kingdom health service.

2 | **The NMC issues guidance on the administration of medicines to doctors and nurses.** ✗

The Nursing and Midwifery Council (NMC) is the professional body for registered nurses and provides guidance on the administration of medicines to all registered nurses across all fields of nursing. The General Medical Council (GMC) is the professional body for doctors.

3 | **When administering a drug, a registered nurse is personally accountable for his or her actions.** ✓

As a professional, you are personally accountable for actions and omissions in your practice and must always be able to justify your actions. Failure to comply with the NMC code regarding the administration of medications may bring your fitness to practise into question and endanger your registration. See www.nmc.org.uk.

4 | **Nurses need a working understanding of medicines administered, therapeutic dosages and side-effects.** ✓

'The administration of medicines is an important aspect of the professional practice of persons whose names are on the Council's register. It is not solely a mechanistic task to be performed in strict compliance with the written prescription of a medical practitioner (can now also be an independent and supplementary prescriber). It requires thought and the exercise of professional judgement ... you must have considered the dosage, weight where appropriate, method of administration, route and timing you must administer or withhold in the context of the patient's condition (for example, Digoxin not usually to be given if pulse below 60) and co-existing therapies, for example, physiotherapy ... you must know the therapeutic uses of the medicine to be administered, its normal dosage, side effects, precautions and contra-indications' (NMC 2007).

5 **Medicines administered by a nursing student must be under the direct supervision of a doctor.**

Nursing students can only administer medicines under the direct supervision of a registered nurse. 'Students must never administer or supply medicinal products without direct supervision' (NMC 2007).

6 **When in use, the medicine trolley must not be left unattended.** ✔

Medicines for use in the ward should be stored in an approved medicine trolley conforming to British Standards. All medicines should be stored according to the manufacturer's recommendations in respect of temperature. Medicine trolleys must be parked when not in use either in a lockable cupboard or attached by lock and chain to the wall or floor. They must never be left unattended when opened. Some hospitals have implemented a policy where drugs are either dispensed directly out of a locked cupboard in a treatment room or dispensed out of a locked cupboard at the patient's bedside. The principles remain the same – that is, the drug storage cupboard must never be left unattended when open.

7 **The pharmacist has the right to audit the medicine cupboard at any time.** ✔

Each pharmacy department has a pharmacist with delegated responsibility for the safe and secure handling of medicines. The pharmacist takes account of statutory requirements and professional guidance and works within specific standard operating procedures (SOPs). The SOPs include provision for checks and spot checks as appropriate. Any discrepancies will be investigated.

8 **A nurse cannot refuse to administer a medicine when the prescription is signed by a doctor.** ✖

A registered nurse can refuse to administer any drug that does not fully meet the NPSA guidelines or where he or she has professional concerns about the drug to be administered. In cases such as this, it is good practice to contact the pharmacist. Remember, the pharmacist has a better working knowledge of drugs than a doctor. It is also good practice to contact the prescriber, so that concerns over the prescription can be shared and further errors can be avoided.

9 **The police will be contacted if there is any suspicion of drug irregularity in any clinical setting.** ✔

In the event of any suspicion of drug irregularities, the hospital authorities will conduct an initial investigation and inform the pharmacy department. It then becomes the responsibility of the pharmacy department to investigate the matter and to contact the police.

10 **Most adverse incidents in hospital are due to drug irregularities.** ✓

The Department of Health defines 'never events' as serious, largely preventable patient safety incidents that should not occur if the available preventative measures have been implemented by healthcare providers. The fact that most adverse incidents in hospital are due to drug irregularities indicates that healthcare professionals are failing to adhere to the correct procedure in relation to the checking and administration of drugs. According to the Department of Health, death or severe harm as a result of administration of the wrong treatment can be attributed in part to nurses and doctors failing to check the patient's identity band. Failure to use standard wristband identification processes means:

- Failure to use patient wristbands that meet the NSPA's design requirements
- Failure to include the four core patient identifiers on wristbands – last name, first name, date of birth and NHS number
- Printing several labels with different patients' details at one time.

MULTIPLE CHOICE

Correct answers identified in bold italics

11 **If a patient has an allergy, the NPSA states this should be:**

a) written on the identity armband only
b) written on the identity armband and verbally reported to colleagues
c) written on the identity armband and on the medicine kardex
d) written on the identity armband, in the patient case notes and the medicine chart

Checking the allergy status of a patient is an absolute requirement and must be documented clearly on the patient's armband, in the case notes and the medicine kardex. In the event that the patient does not have any allergy, this too must be documented. Remember, when asking a patient about allergy status to use language that they can understand; not everyone is aware of what is meant by 'allergy' and you may need to provide examples in order to clarify.

12 **As a nursing student, when checking the patient's identity against the medicine kardex, you should:**

a) bring the kardex with you to the patient and check as per NPSA guidelines

45

b) leave the kardex with the registered nurse and then verbally check the patient's identity as per N P S A guidelines

c) ask the patient to identify themselves and then administer the drug

d) *leave the kardex with the registered nurse and then verbally check the patient's identity and wait for the registered nurse to confirm*

The National Patient Safety Agency has produced a useful set of guidelines for administering oral medications. Checks that should be made include:

- Patient identity
- Allergies
- Consent
- Time
- Route
- Prescription dose.

The N M C guidelines on the administration of medicines refer to the five 'Rs':

- Right patient
- Right route
- Right time
- Right dose
- Right prescription.

13 | If a patient is nil by mouth:

a) all drugs should be withheld

b) all oral drugs should be withheld

c) *the decision to withhold oral drugs should be taken in conjunction with the doctor*

d) if drugs are prescribed, they should be given regardless

The patient will require a risk assessment by the doctor and the decision to withhold or administer a drug will be indicated by: the relevance of the drug to the patient's condition; the risk of adverse effects if the drug was withheld; the risk of adverse effects if the drug was administered.

14 | If a patient has a temporary tracheotomy and is on regular nebulizers, these should be:

a) withheld until the tracheotomy is reversed

b) given via a regular oxygen mask over mouth and nose

c) *given via a tracheotomy mask*

d) given via a non-rebreathing mask over the tracheotomy

Although rare, in some cases the patient will be able to have the drugs via a regular oxygen mask. It is important that you check with the doctor or the specialist nursing team who have expertise in caring for a patient with a tracheotomy.

15 **As a nursing student, when administering a drug, it is:**

a) *never acceptable not to know specific drugs that you are administering*

b) acceptable not to know specific drugs that you are administering as long as the registered nurse knows the drug

c) acceptable not to know the drug you are administering as long as the patient knows the drug

d) acceptable not to know the drug you are administering as long as the carer/relative knows the drug

Nursing students have a responsibility to the patient and the carers/ relatives to know what the medication is, the mode of action of the medication, the normal dosage, any known side-effects, any special precautions the patient needs to take (e.g. avoid sunlight), etc.

16 **If a patient has difficulty swallowing:**

a) all drugs should be withheld

b) *alternate routes should be considered*

c) tablets should be crushed

d) the patient should be persuaded to take a large volume of water to help to swallow medication

Crushing tablets is not recommended, as this can alter the medicine's therapeutic action, making it ineffective or causing adverse effects. If a patient has difficulty swallowing, they are also at risk of aspirating the medication into the lungs. In cases of suspected poor swallow, a swallowing assessment should be requested from the speech and language team. Alternative means of administering the medication must be considered (e.g. liquid form, subcutaneous, intramuscular, intravenous).

17 **If a patient brings his or her own medications into hospital, the medications:**

a) should be taken from the patient and sent to the hospital pharmacy for disposal

b) should be put in the medicine trolley and treated as ward stock

c) should be taken from the patient and sent to the hospital pharmacy for storage *d)* are the property of the patient to whom they were supplied and must not be taken without consent

A doctor, nurse and/or pharmacist should make specific enquiries to determine whether the patient is taking any prescribed medicines or any other medicinal preparations and whether the patient has brought them into hospital. The patient should, however, be asked to surrender, for examination by a doctor, nurse or pharmacist, any such medicines or other preparations brought to the hospital.

18 **The deltoid muscle should be used when:**

a) a slow uptake of the medication is required

b) a fast uptake of the medication is required

c) 4–5 millilitres of medication are to be given

d) 10 millilitres of medication are to be given

The gluteus maximus muscle has the slowest uptake of medication, whereas the deltoid has the fastest. Only 1–2 millilitres can be administered into the deltoid muscle.

19 **Needles are colour-coded according to their gauge. When administrating an intramuscular injection, it is generally acceptable to use:**

a) a blue needle   b) an orange needle   c) a grey needle   *d) a green needle*

Needles are colour-coded according to their gauge (G); the higher the gauge, the narrower the lumen of the needle:

- Green: 21 G and 38 mm long

- Blue: 23 G and 25 mm long

- Orange: 25 G and 10 mm long

- Grey: 27 G and 16 mm or 25 mm long

FILL IN THE BLANKS

20 A subcutaneous (SC) injection means a drug is given beneath the _skin_ into the connective tissue or _fat_ immediately underlying the _dermis_.

21 Intramuscular (IM) administration means a drug is injected into _skeletal muscle_. Absorption occurs more _rapidly_ than with SC injection because of greater tissue blood flow.

22 | The intravenous route is an injection directly into the *bloodstream* and produces an immediate response.

This is because the absorption process is circumvented. Intravenous drugs should always be administered slowly and by a nurse/doctor who is competent to give such drugs.

23 | Epidural administration of a drug means that it is injected via a small catheter into the *epidural* space.

The epidural space is the space outside of the dura mater of the spinal cord. This route is increasingly being used to administer opioids for pain management.

24 | As a drug enters the bloodstream, it binds to protein, mainly *albumin*.

The drug forms a drug-protein complex. The process can be reversed.

25 | The factors influencing drug-protein binding are the degree of drug binding, the competition for binding sites and *hypoalbuminaemia*.

Low levels of albumin in the blood are known as hypoalbuminaemia and may be caused by malnutrition or hepatic (liver) damage. If a patient with hypoalbuminaemia is administered a drug that has plasma protein binding, more of the free form of the drug circulates, resulting in a greater risk of overdosage and toxicity.

26 | The process of chemically inactivating a drug by converting it into a more water-soluble compound or metabolite is known as *metabolism*.

Metabolism is the method used by the body to produce homeostasis and involves a balance between the synthesis of chemicals and their breakdown. The principle metabolic organ in the body is the liver and the liver plays a huge part in the metabolism of most drugs.

27 | *Children* with immature metabolizing systems and *older adults* with degenerative enzyme function experience depressed metabolism.

These groups have greater difficulty in breaking down drugs and are therefore at risk of accidental drug overdose. It is therefore important that extra care is taken when prescribing and administering drugs to these vulnerable groups.

28 | The *liver* is a major metabolizing organ for drugs.

The process of chemically inactivating a drug by converting it into a more soluble metabolite that can be excreted by the body is carried out by the liver.

29 **Abnormal clearance of a drug may be anticipated when a client has *renal* function impairment.**

Creatinine clearance is a useful indicator of renal function and is based on the collection of a 24-hour urine specimen. However, such specimen collection is often inaccurate because of the loss of some of the patient's urine. Serum creatinine blood results are used instead.

Nutrition and fluid balance

INTRODUCTION

The importance of good nutrition and fluid balance cannot be underestimated. The role of balanced nutrition and fluids in influencing the recovery from illness and disability is not in dispute. Whatever problems your patient is presenting with, and whether it is to prevent complications or to promote recovery, food and fluids play a vital role in contributing to health. The Department of Health recommends that all staff providing any nutritional care have appropriate skills and training and should be regularly updated on such matters.

Malnutrition may be a cause or a consequence of ill health. Malnourished patients are more likely to develop complications both mentally and physically, which in turn can lead to prolonged hospital stays and higher mortality rates than their counterparts receiving good nutrition.

As a healthcare professional, it is your responsibility to ensure that you have a sound working knowledge of the effects of nutrition and fluids on your patients' health. Nurses must be able to identify patients at risk and take the appropriate steps to improve their nutritional status. It is the responsibility of every nurse to challenge poor practice in relation to nutrition and hydration and take the lead in providing good nutritional care planning. In spite of this, the National Institute for Health and Clinical Excellence (NICE) has identified that the existing knowledge of nutrition among healthcare professionals is poor.

Useful resources

British Association for Parenteral and Enteral Nutrition (UK):
http://www.bapen.org.uk

National Institute for Health & Clinical Excellence:
http://www.nice.org.uk

NHS National Patient Safety Agency:
http://www.npsa.nhs.uk

Nurses! Test yourself in Anatomy & Physiology Chapter 9

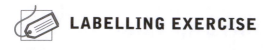

LABELLING EXERCISE

1–15   Identify the components of the digestive system in Figure 4.1, using the terms provided in the box:

Figure 4.1 The digestive system

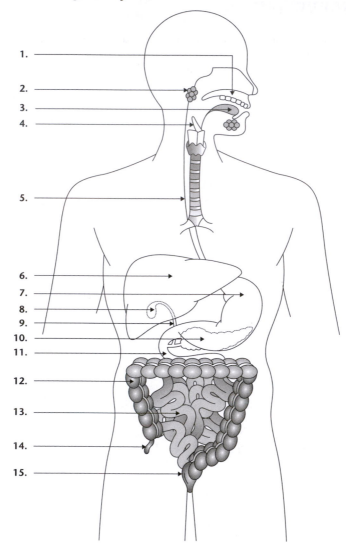

teeth

tongue

epiglottis

oesophagus

liver

stomach

gall bladder

duodenum

common bile duct

pancreas

large intestine

small intestine

appendix

rectum

salivary gland

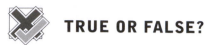 **TRUE OR FALSE?**

Are the following statements true or false?

16   Percutaneous endoscopic gastrostomy (PEG) is a type of parenteral nutrition.

17   BMI stands for Body Measurement Index.

18   A pH of less than 5.5 is consistent with gastric placement.

19   Patients receiving nutrition via a PEG or nasogastric (NG) tube do not require oral hygiene.

20   Parenteral nutrition is the administration of pre-digested nutrients directly into the bloodstream via an IV line.

21   Patients receiving parenteral nutrition must have their temperature recorded at least every 4 hours.

22   When receiving parenteral nutrition, blood glucose monitoring should be carried out daily.

23   If an enteral solution ('feed') is running behind schedule, the infusion rate should be increased accordingly.

24   Enteral nutrition means feeding a patient into a vein.

25 A nasogastric tube is inserted via one of the nostrils, down the nasopharynx and into the stomach.

26 When passing an NG tube, it is recommended to encourage the patient to swallow to keep the epiglottis open.

27 When receiving feeds via the PEG tube, the patient must be strictly nil orally.

a b c d MULTIPLE CHOICE

Identify one correct answer for each of the following.

28 How much does a litre of fluid weigh approximately?

a) 500 grams

b) 750 grams

c) 1 kilogram

d) 1.2 kilograms

29 The recommended periods of fasting pre-operatively are:

a) 2 hours from clear fluids and 4 hours from solids

b) 2 hours from clear fluids and 6 hours from solids

c) 2 hours from clear fluids, 4 hours from milky fluids and 6 hours from solids

d) 4 hours from fluids and 6 hours from solids

30 The term used to describe difficulty in swallowing is:

a) dysphagia

b) dyspepsia

c) dysphasia

d) dyspnoea

31 Obesity is classified as having a body mass index (BMI) greater than:

a) 18.5

b) 24.9

c) 29.9

d) 34.9

32 Anthropometric measurements include:

a) height

b) weight

c) triceps skinfold thickness

d) diameter of dominant wrist

33 Subjective nutritional assessment includes:

a) BMI

b) serum albumin levels

c) 24-hour urine collection

d) appetite

34 To ascertain correct placement of an NG tube, it is advisable to use:

a) litmus paper

b) pH graded paper

c) 'whoosh' test

d) a test feed

35 If you are unable to obtain aspirate from the NG tube in an unconscious patient, you may:

a) go ahead and feed as prescribed

b) insert water down the tube

c) change the patient's position to alternative side and try again to get aspirate in 1 hour

d) sit patient upright and attempt to get aspirate again

36 Aspiration should not take place after a feed until:

a) 15 minutes have passed

b) 30 minutes have passed

c) 45 minutes have passed

d) 1 hour has passed

37 The patient will require a further nutritional assessment if their MUST score is higher than:

a) 1

b) 2

c) 3

d) 4

38 Immediately before and after administrating feed or medication via a PEG tube, it is important to:

a) flush tube with 30/60 millilitres of water

b) aspirate tube

c) insert 30/60 millilitres volume of air

d) flush tube with 30/60 millilitres of normal saline

39 The length of the NG tube to be inserted is determined by assessing:

a) the patient's height

b) the patient's weight

c) the total distance from the top of the client's nose to ear lobe and then to the tip of the xiphoid process

d) the total distance from the top of the client's head to the tip of the xiphoid process

FILL IN THE BLANKS

Fill in the blanks in each statement using the words in the box below.
Not all of them are required, so choose carefully.

malnutrition	pressure sores
increased respiratory rate	bulimia
anorexia	impaired wound healing
pyrexia	hypothermia
pale	swollen
spongy	poor cough pressure
pain relief	oral hygiene
hand washing	utensils
comfortable	salt
supine	exercise
toileting	preference
safe temperature	allergy
nutritional	refeeding
fluid	dumping
electrolyte	urea
blood glucose	parenteral
enteral	72 hours
positive	

40 _____ has a detrimental effect on physical and psychological function.

41 The gums of a person with malnutrition can appear _____ and _____.

42 The patient suffering with malnutrition may have impaired thermo-regulation, which could lead to _____.

43 A chest infection can be a consequence of malnutrition due to _____.

44 Comfort measures such as _____, _____ and _____ should be provided prior to mealtimes to encourage appetite. Encouraging or providing _____ prior to mealtimes helps improve the patient's ability to taste the food. The food provided should be of the patient's _____ and must be at a _____. To promote independence, the patient should be assisted to a _____ position so they can reach the food easily and the appropriate _____ should be provided.

45 Before commencing enteral nutrition, the patient's _____ status to any food in the formula should be checked. The patient's _____ balance must be accurately recorded.

46 _____ and _____ & _____ balance should be closely monitored, especially in patients receiving _____ nutrition, as disturbances in these levels may be indicative of _____ syndrome.

47 Calculate Mrs Brown's fluid balance from the table below:

Oral intake	IV input	Output	
240 mL water	2000 mL NaCl	2150 mL urine	100 mL surgical drain
600 mL tea			
Total intake =		Total output =	

48 Mrs. Brown has a _____ fluid balance.

49 When administering clear solutions, an IV giving set should usually be changed every _____.

ANSWERS

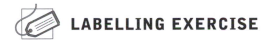

LABELLING EXERCISE

Figure 4.2 The digestive system

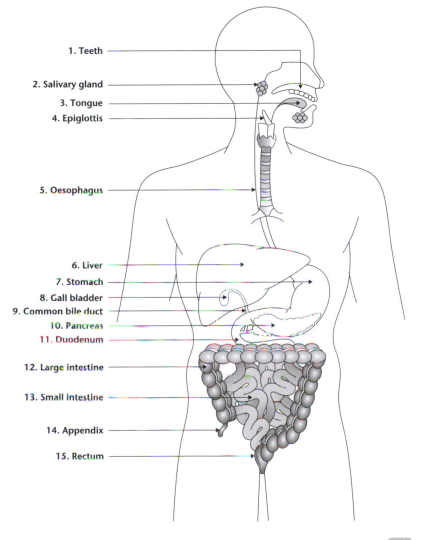

1. Teeth
2. Salivary gland
3. Tongue
4. Epiglottis
5. Oesophagus
6. Liver
7. Stomach
8. Gall bladder
9. Common bile duct
10. Pancreas
11. Duodenum
12. Large intestine
13. Small intestine
14. Appendix
15. Rectum

Teeth: The strongest stuff in the body! Their purpose is to rip, grind and mash all the food we put into our mouths.

 Salivary gland: Three main salivary glands deliver their juices, saliva, into the mouth. This fluid enzyme helps to soften up the food, the first chemical action along the digestive tract.

 Tongue: One very strong muscle made for rolling food around the mouth so the teeth can perform best. It also has taste buds: sensors of sweet, sour, salty and bitter tastes.

4 **Epiglottis:** This 'trap door' belongs to both the respiratory system and the digestive system. Swallowing triggers closing of the epiglottis over the trachea to prevent food and fluids from entering our lungs.

5 **Oesophagus:** A muscular canal running from the pharynx to the stomach. The tongue pushes a 'bolus' of food into the oesophagus to start it on its way to the stomach. 'Peristalsis' is the name used to describe the rhythmic contract and release actions of this muscle and most all others along the digestive tract.

6 **Liver:** One of the 'accessory' organs of digestion. Food doesn't actually pass through this organ. Instead, this organ secretes bile that is passed along to the gall bladder for concentration and storage.

7 **Stomach:** Most food that we eat becomes unrecognizable here in the stomach. Gastric acids are triggered by the presence of food that turns the food into a thick soup-like substance called chyme.

8 **Gall bladder:** Another accessory organ; food doesn't touch this one either. It is a pear-shaped sac about 10 cm long and is the reservoir for bile. Concentrated bile is released into the duodenum as needed to break down fats into an absorbable form.

9 **Common bile duct:** This duct carries bile from the gall bladder and liver into the duodenum (upper part of the small intestine) of the small bowel.

10 **Pancreas:** Helps control the body's sugar. If your blood sugar gets too high, insulin is released to counteract it. If your sugars are low, glucagon is released into the bloodstream. Both insulin and glucagon are produced by the pancreas.

11 **Duodenum:** The duodenum is the first section of the 6.5-metre-long small intestine. It starts at the pyloric sphincter of the stomach and runs about 25 cm The duodenum is largely responsible for the continuing breaking-down process of food, with the jejunum and ileum mainly responsible for the transfer of nutrients into the bloodstream.

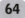

Large intestine: There are many sections to the large intestine – the appendix, caecum, ascending (rising) colon, transverse (across) colon, descending (going down) colon, sigmoid colon, rectum and anus. The main purpose of the large intestine is to pass remaining essential nutrients into the bloodstream, and store and eliminate waste leftovers. As the nutritional fluids are absorbed and transferred out to the bloodstream, the contents become more solid and compact.

 Small intestine: The small bowel has three main sections: the duodenum, jejunum and ileum. The duodenum is responsible for continuing to break down food into liquid form and the jejunum and ileum for absorption of nutrients into the bloodstream. The mostly digested contents continue to be transformed into faeces as they are moved along by peristalsis.

 Appendix: Little is understood about this little worm-like structure that extends from the first section of the large intestine. Sometimes a piece of food gets stuck in here causing an infection.

 Rectum: The last portion of the large intestine used for storage of faeces ready for disposal. When the rectum becomes full, it triggers nerves that carry that message to the brain.

 ## TRUE OR FALSE?

 Percutaneous endoscopic gastrostomy (PEG) is a type of parenteral nutrition.

PEG feeding is a type of enteral feed, i.e. fed into the gastro-intestinal system. Enteral feeding is chosen when the patient is unable to ingest any or sufficient food to meet their nutritional needs and/or if the upper gastro-intestinal tract is impaired.

 BMI stands for Body Measurement Index.

BMI stands for Body Mass Index (see answer to Question 31).

A pH of less than 5.5 is consistent with gastric placement.

Gastric aspirate tends to be acidic and have a pH of 1–4 but may be as high as 6 in some patients on medication to control gastric secretions.

29 **The recommended periods of fasting pre-operatively are:**

a) 2 hours from clear fluids and 4 hours from solids
b) 2 hours from clear fluids and 6 hours from solids
c) 2 hours from clear fluids, 4 hours from milky fluids and 6 hours from solids
d) 4 hours from fluids and 6 hours from solids

Patients undergoing surgery are at risk of aspiration. During anaesthesia, the swallow reflex is suppressed. There is a risk of the stomach contents being inhaled into the lungs. Certain groups of patients, such as older adults or those suffering from diabetes, are at a higher risk. Fasting from food and fluids can minimize risk. Pre-operative fasting in adults undergoing elective surgery is 'the 2 and 6 rule'. The anaesthetic team should consider further interventions in high-risk groups. Despite this evidence, many patients are still fasted for long periods leading to preventable complications.

30 **The term used to describe difficulty in swallowing is:**

a) dysphagia   b) dyspepsia   c) dysphasia   d) dyspnoea

Dysphagia is the term used to describe any impairment of eating, drinking and swallowing. It is a symptom of other underlying pathology rather than a disease. If not diagnosed, it can lead to nutritional compromise and other health-related problems. If suspected, a full assessment using a multidisciplinary approach is required. People with dysphagia can present with obvious and less obvious indicators of the problem. For example, difficulty swallowing, drooling, coughing and choking before, during or after swallowing may be present. On the other hand, less obvious signs may be present, such as recurrent chest infections, changes in respiratory pattern or unexplained temperature spikes.

31 **Obesity is classified as having a body mass index (BMI) greater than:**

a) 18.5   b) 24.9   *c) 29.9*   d) 34.9

A healthy BMI is from 18.5 to 24.9. Overweight is classified as a BMI of 25 to 29.9, 30 to 39.9 is considered obese and a BMI greater than 40 is referred to as morbidly obese. The key disadvantage of BMI is that it assumes that excess weight is a result of excess fat and doesn't account for other reasons such as oedema or large muscle mass, so a very muscular person could fall into the obese or even very obese range. Different reference charts are used for adults and children. All measurements falling outside the normal range indicate a patient with a greater health risk and further nutritional needs must be assessed accordingly.

32 **Anthropometric measurements include:**

a) height   b) weight   *c) triceps skinfold thickness*
d) diameter of dominant wrist

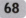

Following a nutritional screening that identifies a person at risk, it is necessary to carry out a further, more comprehensive assessment. Part of this assessment may include anthropometric arm measurements; these are measurements that provide information about the body composition being made up of fat or muscle. There are three different measurements that make up anthropometric measurements:

- triceps skinfold measurements
- mid-arm circumference
- mid-arm muscle circumference.

These are all quite intricate measures and require specific training for them to be carried out accurately. Skinfold measurement requires three readings to be taken and an average of the three to be recorded. While the triceps skinfold is the most commonly used, a skinfold measurement may be taken from any appropriate site, including the biceps, calf, thigh, subscapular or suprailiac skinfolds. Special skinfold callipers are used to measure to the nearest millimetre. Values recorded are compared with standard reference measurements: less than or more than 90% of the reference value indicates less than average or more than average fat reserves.

33 Subjective nutritional assessment includes:

a) **BMI**   b) serum albumin levels   c) 24-hour urine collection
d) appetite

Nutritional assessment includes subjective, objective and laboratory data. Serum albumin levels and 24-hour urine collection are examples of laboratory data; appetite is an example of objective data; and BMI is a subjective assessment. BMI measures weight in relationship to height and is calculated using centimetres and kilograms. The formula for calculating BMI is as follows:

$$BMI = \frac{\text{weight in kilograms}}{(\text{height in metres}) \times (\text{height in metres})}$$

34 To ascertain correct placement of an NG tube, it is advisable to use:

a) litmus paper   *b) pH graded paper*   c) 'whoosh' test   d) a test feed

Aspirate tube and check secretions. Measure pH using pH paper not litmus paper. It is recommended that a pH < 5.5 is consistent with gastric placement. Small-bore tubes can be harder to aspirate. Routine X-ray is not recommended – local policy exists for high-risk groups, e.g. intensive care or confused patients.

35 If you are unable to obtain aspirate from the NG tube in an unconscious patient, you may:

a) go ahead and feed as prescribed
b) insert water down the tube

    c) change the patient's position to alternative side and try again to get aspirate in 1 hour

    d) sit patient upright and attempt to get aspirate again

Position of NG tube should be verified on initial placement, before each feed or if it becomes dislodged. If aspirate cannot be obtained or the pH is > 5.5, feeding should not be commenced. It is recommended that the patient's position is changed and the aspirate rechecked in one hour.

36 | **Aspiration should not take place after a feed until:**

a) 15 minutes have passed   b) 30 minutes have passed

c) 45 minutes have passed   *d) 1 hour has passed*

The feed can increase the stomach pH, so it is recommended that aspiration should take place at least one hour after the feed has stopped.

37 | **The patient will require a further nutritional assessment if their MUST score is higher than:**

a) 1   b) 2   c) 3   d) 4

The Malnutrition Universal Screening Tool (MUST) was developed by the British Association for Parenteral and Enteral Nutrition (BAPEN). It is a five-step screening tool to identify adults who are malnourished or at risk of malnutrition, and is designed to be used by all care workers across all care settings. The MUST includes management guidelines that can be used to develop a plan of care as appropriate to the patient's needs. A score of 0 is low risk and repeated screenings according to the care setting are to be carried out. A score of 1 is taken as medium risk and observation of dietary intake along with repeated screenings according to the care setting is recommended. If the MUST score is 2 or above, the patient should be referred to a dietician for a more comprehensive nutritional assessment.

38 | **Immediately before and after administrating feed or medication via a PEG tube, it is important to:**

    a) flush tube with 30/60 millilitres of water

    b) aspirate tube

    c) insert 30/60 millilitres volume of air

    d) flush tube with 30/60 millilitres of normal saline

To maintain patency, it is important to flush the tube before and after administration of feeds or medication. Normally tap water is acceptable; however, if your patient is immune-compromised, sterile water is recommended; if the patient is at home, they may use boiled and cooled water.

39 **The length of the NG tube to be inserted is determined by assessing:**

a) the patient's height   b) the patient's weight

c) *the total distance from the top of the patient's nose to ear lobe and then to the tip of the xiphoid process*

d) the total distance from the top of the patient's head to the tip of the xiphoid process

Determine how far to insert the tube. Use the tube to measure from the tip of the nose to the tip of ear lobe and then from earlobe to the tip of the xiphoid process.

FILL IN THE BLANKS

40 *Malnutrition* **has a detrimental effect on physical and psychological function.**

Malnutrition is defined as 'a state of nutrition in which a deficiency, excess or imbalance of energy protein and other nutrients causes measurable adverse effects on tissues/body form (body shape, size, composition) and function and clinical outcome'. Malnutrition can affect every system and tissue of the body. The physical, psychological and social implications of malnutrition are well documented. It is a major public health issue, the prevention and management of which have become an important aspect of the nurse's role. Vitamin C deficiency causes spongy, swollen, inflamed gums that bleed easily. Malnutrition causes hypothermia, which can put patients at risk of a fall, especially the elderly.

41 **The gums of a person with malnutrition can appear** *spongy* **and** *swollen*.

Vitamin C deficiency causes spongy swollen inflamed gums that bleed easily. Care should be taken when performing mouth care on patients who suffer from malnutrition.

42 **The patient suffering with malnutrition may have impaired thermoregulation, which could lead to** *hypothermia*.

Malnutrition causes hypothermia which can put patients, especially older adults, at risk of fall. Hypothermia is a condition in which the core body temperature is 35°C or less.

43 **A chest infection can be a consequence of malnutrition due to _poor cough pressure_.**

Patients who are malnourished often become easily fatigued. A poor cough pressure can predispose the patient to chest infections. Inactivity and weakness are also contributing factors. When patients do develop a chest infection, recovery can be slow, leading to longer periods in hospital and the potential to develop other complications.

44 **Comfort measures such as _pain relief, toileting_ and _hand washing_ should be provided prior to mealtimes to encourage appetite. Encouraging or providing _oral hygiene_ prior to mealtimes helps improve the patient's ability to taste the food. The food provided should be of the patient's _preference_ and must be at a _safe temperature_. To promote independence, the patient should be assisted to a _comfortable_ position so they can reach the food easily and the appropriate _utensils_ should be provided.**

To promote the optimum environment for eating and drinking, it is important that the patient is comfortable and in an environment free from distractions. The temperature of the food is another factor that affects appetite, so it important to provide hot and cold foods at the correct temperature; foods that are too hot might cause injury. Adapted cutlery, plates and non-slip mats should be appropriate and easily cleaned. Assisting a patient with eating and drinking requires considerable skill and its importance must never be underestimated.

45 **Before commencing enteral nutrition, the patient's _allergy_ status to any food in the formula should be checked. The patient's _fluid_ balance must be accurately recorded.**

46 **_Blood glucose_ and _urea_ & _electrolyte_ balance should be closely monitored, especially in patients receiving _parenteral_ nutrition, as disturbances in these levels may be indicative of _refeeding_ syndrome.**

As with all medications, an allergy check is important. Common allergies include milk, sugar and eggs. At all times it is important to record intake accurately. Refeeding syndrome is a metabolic complication; a person who has had very little food for more than 5 days is at high risk. The sudden introduction of infused nutrients causes a change in the metabolism of the fats and carbohydrates; this in turn can cause major electrolyte imbalance and the key way of detecting this is through close clinical and biochemical monitoring.

47 | **Calculate Mrs Brown's fluid balance from the table below:**

Oral intake	IV input	Output	
240 mL water	2000 mL NaCl	2150 mL urine	100 mL surgical drain
600 mL tea			
Total intake = **2840 mL**		Total output = **2250 mL**	

48 | **Mrs Brown has a _positive_ fluid balance.**

49 | **When administering clear solutions, an IV giving set should usually be changed every _72 hours_.**

Mrs Brown has a positive fluid balance, which means that she has a greater intake than output; had the output been greater than the input, it would be referred to as a negative fluid balance. Changing of giving sets should be performed according to local policy; however, they must be changed at least every 72 hours.include milk, sugar and eggs. At all times it is important to record intake accurately. Refeeding syndrome is a metabolic complication; a person who has had very little food for more than 5 days is at high risk. The sudden introduction of infused nutrients causes a change in the metabolism of the fats and carbohydrates; this in turn can cause major electrolyte imbalance and the key way of detecting this is through close clinical and biochemical monitoring.

5 Elimination skills

INTRODUCTION

Elimination of urine and faeces is essential to the normal function of the human body. The ability to eliminate can be affected by the physiology of ageing, disease process, medications, chemotherapy, surgery, disability and mental health problems. When something goes wrong and an individual cannot attend to their elimination needs, they become dependent on a nurse to provide this most intimate of care. As such, you will be expected not only to provide the nursing care but also to understand the rationale for the care provided. Caring for a patient who has problems associated with elimination is one of the most personal and sensitive duties a nurse can engage in for a fellow human being.

To provide nursing care for someone with elimination problems you must understand the principles of normal elimination patterns, the assessment tools employed and appropriate nursing interventions. This chapter seeks to test your knowledge of skills associated with elimination.

Useful resources

The Royal Marsden Hospital Manual of Clinical Nursing Procedures

Essential Nursing Skills

Nurses! Test Yourself in Anatomy and Physiology
Chapters 9 and 10

Nurses! Test Yourself in Pathophysiology
Chapters 9 and 10

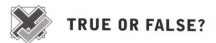 **TRUE OR FALSE?**

Are the following statements true or false?

 1 The normal frequency of bowel movement in the population varies from once every three days to three times a day.

 2 Misconceptions about bowel habits have led to excessive laxative use.

 3 Where possible, constipation should be treated with drugs.

 4 More fluids and fibre in the diet can often relieve constipation.

 5 All episodes of diarrhoea should be considered non-infectious until bacteriology results are received.

 6 The prevention and/or correction of dehydration is the first step in managing an episode of diarrhoea.

7 Catheter-associated infections account for 35–40% of hospital infections.

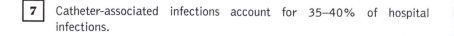 **8** A three-way Foley catheter is most commonly used for patients who require short-term bladder drainage.

9   Urine is typically clear, pale to deep yellow in colour and slightly alkaline (pH >7).

10   Leucocyte esterase is not normally found in urine and is an indicator of infection.

MULTIPLE CHOICE

Identify one correct answer for each of the following.

11 Constipation is defined as:

a) an abnormal increase in the quantity and frequency of stool
b) delayed movement of intestinal content through the bowel
c) inflammatory disorder affecting the small bowel
d) inflammatory disorder affecting the large bowel

12 A laxative that works by increasing the stool mass and stimulating peristalsis is categorized as:

a) a faecal softener
b) an osmotic laxative
c) a bulk-forming drug
d) a stimulant laxative

13 Senna is an example of:

a) a faecal softener
b) a bulking agent
c) an osmotic laxative
d) a stimulant laxative

14 Diarrhoea is defined as:

a) an abnormal increase in the quantity of stool
b) an abnormal increase in the quantity and frequency of stool
c) an abnormal increase in the quantity, frequency and fluid content of stool and associated with urgency, perianal discomfort and incontinence
d) more than one stool per day

15 Stools can be graded using a stool chart such as:

a) the Bristol stool chart

b) the Brighton stool chart

c) the Braden stool chart

d) the Birmingham stool chart

16 Skin care is particularly important with diarrhoea since it contains:

a) high levels of fat

b) high levels of enzymes

c) high levels of water

d) high levels of laxatives

17 When administrating an enema, the patient should be instructed to:

a) lie on the right side with knees flexed

b) lie on the left side with knees flexed

c) lie on back with knees flexed

d) lie on left side with legs straight

18 When administrating suppositories, the patient should be instructed to:

a) retain the suppository for at least 20 minutes or as long as possible

b) 'bear down' as if defecating

c) retain the suppository for a maximum of 5 minutes

d) expel the suppository immediately

19 A specimen of urine from a patient with a urinary catheter should be:

a) obtained from the urinary bag by draining urine from the exit port

b) obtained from the sampling ports using an aseptic technique

c) obtained from any part of the catheter

d) obtained by removing the catheter and requesting the patient to void into a sterile dish

20 The urinary catheter balloon should be inflated using:

a) air

b) tap water

c) sterile water

d) 0.9% sodium chloride

21 Presence of blood in the urine is defined as:

a) haematemesis

b) haemoptysis

c) haematuria

d) haematocrit

22 When collecting a catheter specimen of urine (CSU), if there is no urine present in the catheter tubing:

a) clamp the catheter to allow urine to collect

b) take a sample from the catheter bag

c) clamp the tubing below the sample port until sufficient urine collects

d) disconnect the catheter to collect the specimen

FILL IN THE BLANKS

Fill in the blanks in each statement using the words in the box below.
Not all of them are required, so choose carefully.

urinary tract infection	fibre
alkaline	bulk
closed circuit	peristalsis
bacteria	green
fungi	exercise
viruses	diet
fluid	defecate
paralytic ileus	colonic obstruction
motility	mucosa
acidic	vitamins

23 Catheterizing patients places them in significant danger of acquiring a
_____ .

24 Urine is normally _____ .

25 An indwelling catheter used in conjunction with an attached collection
bag is known as a _____ .

26 Acute diarrhoea is usually caused by _____ and/or _____ .

27 Increasing dietary _____ increases stool _____ , which in turn improves _____ and stool transit time.

28 Individuals who suffer from constipation should be encouraged to increase their amount of _____.

29 The primary causes of constipation are inadequate diet, poor _____ intake, lifestyle change, ignoring the urge to _____.

30 Enemas are contraindicated in _____ and _____.

31 Stimulant laxatives increase intestinal _____ by direct action on the _____.

32 Put the following 10 steps for doing a urinalysis using a reagent strip in the correct sequence.

	Obtain a specimen of fresh urine from the patient
	Wait the required time interval before reading the strip agent against the chart on the bottle
	Wash and dry hands and put on gloves and apron
	Document urinalysis reading and inform nurse in charge and medical staff of any abnormalities
	Hold the reagent stick at an angle
	Explain the procedure to the patient
	Dispose of urine sample in either the sluice or toilet
	Dip the reagent stick into the urine. The strip should be completely immersed and then removed. Tap edge of strip gently along the container to remove excess urine
	Check that the reagent sticks are in date
	Remove apron and gloves and wash and dry hands

ANSWERS

TRUE OR FALSE?

1 | **The normal frequency of bowel movement in the population varies from once every three days to three times a day.** ✓

It is thought that less than 10% of the population has a bowel evacuation daily. The stimulus to defecate is initiated by the response to faeces entering the rectum. This reflex encourages the internal anal sphincter muscle to relax, the desire to defecate being conveyed to the brain and interpreted by the individual as an awareness of the requirement to eliminate faeces.

2 | **Misconceptions about bowel habits have led to excessive laxative use.** ✓

The myth of a daily bowel evacuation has resulted in laxative abuse becoming one of the most common types of drug abuse in the Western World. Constipation is practically unheard of in, for example, the African countries and can be attributed to poor diet and lack of exercise in more developed countries.

3 | **Where possible, constipation should be treated with drugs.**

After an initial assessment, constipation should be treated through education and lifestyle changes before resorting to drugs. The individual should be encouraged to engage in more physical activity and to increase fluid intake. The physical activity will increase the motility of the gastro-intestinal tract and the fluid will assist with softening the bowel content. Laxatives should generally be avoided except where straining will exacerbate a condition (such as angina) or increase the risk of bleeding as in haemorrhoids.

4 | **More fluids and fibre in the diet can often relieve constipation.** ✓

Fibre increases the bulk in the large bowel and thus aids peristalsis. Fluid helps to dilute the bowel content and therefore makes transition easier. The individual's fluid intake should be assessed, the target being an intake of 30–35 mL/kg per day.

5 | **All episodes of diarrhoea should be considered non-infectious until bacteriology results are received.**

Diarrhoea should always be treated as potentially infectious until proved otherwise. This will require all healthcare workers to adopt universal precautions and wear gloves and aprons, and nurse the patient in isolation.

6 | **The prevention and/or correction of dehydration is the first step in managing an episode of diarrhoea.** ✔

Episodes of diarrhoea can cause the patient to lose large quantities of body fluid and lead to dehydration. Dehydration is potentially life-threatening and must be prevented or detected early and managed with drinks or intravenous fluids as appropriate. Remember it is not just fluid that is lost but also electrolytes!

7 | **Catheter-associated infections account for 35–40% of hospital infections.**

Catheterizing patients puts them in significant danger of acquiring a urinary tract infection and the longer the catheter is in place, the greater the danger. Secondary complications associated with urinary tract infection include encrustation and blockage and bypassing. Catheterization is best avoided if at all possible.

8 | **A three-way Foley catheter is most commonly used for patients who require short-term bladder drainage.** ✖

A two-way Foley catheter is most commonly used; there are two channels, one for drainage and one for inflating the balloon. The insertion of a urinary catheter requires an aseptic technique. A three-way catheter is normally used to introduce fluids into the bladder for irrigation purposes.

9 | **Urine is typically clear, pale to deep yellow in colour and slightly alkaline (pH >7).** ✖

Urine is formed in the renal tubules and enters the collecting ducts, which empty urine into the kidney calyx. When urine collects in the renal pelvis, it flows to the bladder. The plasma that is filtered into the renal tubule contains water, glucose, electrolytes and nitrogenous wastes. The excess fluid is removed in the filtration process along with acid waste products (urea, creatinine, hydrogen ions) in the form of urine. Urine is therefore slightly acidic (pH 6) and is typically clear, pale to deep yellow in colour.

10 | **Leucocyte esterase is not normally found in urine and is an indicator of infection.** ✔

Leucocyte esterase in urine is an indicator of bacterial infection. A culture should be performed to identify the organism and determine antibiotic sensitivity. Urinary infection, like any other bacterial infection, is associated with an increased number of leucocytes and an inflammatory response that results in the production of pus. The urine presents as cloudy when pus is present and it can be foul-smelling.

MULTIPLE CHOICE

Correct answers identified in bold italics

11 **Constipation is defined as:**

a) an abnormal increase in the quantity and frequency of stool
b)　delayed movement of intestinal content through the bowel
c) inflammatory disorder affecting the small bowel
d) inflammatory disorder affecting the large bowel

Constipation results in delayed evacuation of the bowel due to decreased motility of the intestines. The stools are difficult to pass and are usually hard and lumpy in appearance and the longer the faeces remain in the intestine, the more water is absorbed from them, and the harder and drier they become. The effective treatment is dependent on a thorough assessment.

12 **A laxative that works by increasing the stool mass and stimulating peristalsis is categorized as:**

a) a faecal softener　　b) an osmotic laxative　　*c) a bulk-forming drug*
d) a stimulant laxative

These drugs must be taken with plenty of fluids to avoid intestinal obstruction. They may take up to three days to be effective. Bulk-forming laxatives relieve constipation by increasing faecal mass, which stimulates peristalsis. Unprocessed wheat bran, taken with food or fruit juice, is a most effective bulk-forming preparation.

13 **Senna is an example of:**

a) a faecal softener　　b) a bulking agent　　c) an osmotic laxative
d) a stimulant laxative

Stimulant laxatives increase motility by direct stimulant action on the mucosa. They usually act 12 hours after oral administration and within one hour if given as a suppository. Stimulant laxatives often cause abdominal cramping and prolonged use may lead to impaired bowel function. Stimulant laxatives include bisacodyl, senna and dantron. Prolonged use of stimulant laxatives can cause diarrhoea and other complications such as hypokalaemia.

14 **Diarrhoea is defined as:**

a) an abnormal increase in the quantity of stool
b) an abnormal increase in the quantity and frequency of stool
c) an abnormal increase in the quantity, frequency and fluid content of stool and associated with urgency, perianal discomfort and incontinence

d) more than one stool per day

Diarrhoea is classified as either acute or chronic. Acute diarrhoea usually lasts less than two weeks and could be associated with, for example, drug therapies such as antibiotics or chemotherapy. Chronic diarrhoea, on the other hand, normally lasts longer than two weeks and can be associated with chronic conditions, such as inflammatory bowel disease, diverticulitis or neoplasms.

15 **Stools can be graded using a stool chart such as:**

a) the Bristol stool chart b) the Brighton stool chart c) the Braden stool chart d) the Birmingham stool chart

The Bristol stool chart is an aid to classification of stool according to form. Other factors to be considered when assessing a stool include colour, consistency and odour. For example, *Clostridium difficile* (antibiotic-associated colitis caused by colonization of the colon with *C. difficile*, which may follow antibiotic therapy) has a distinctive odour.

16 **Skin care is particularly important with diarrhoea since it contains:**

a) high levels of fat *b) high levels of enzymes* c) high levels of water
d) high levels of laxatives

Diarrhoea has high levels of faecal enzymes that come into contact with the perianal skin and the area requires cleansing with warm water immediately after each episode of diarrhoea. Failure to clean the perianal area adequately may result in skin excoriation and skin breakdown.

17 **When administrating an enema, the patient should be instructed to:**

a) lie on the right side with knees flexed
b) lie on the left side with knees flexed
c) lie on back with knees flexed
d) lie on left side with legs straight

By laying the patient on the left side, the suppository is easier to pass into the rectum as it will be following the natural anatomy of the colon. Flexing the knees will help to ease any discomfort as the suppository passes via the anal sphincter.

18 **When administrating suppositories, the patient should be instructed to:**

a) retain the suppository for at least 20 minutes or as long as possible
b) 'bear down' as if defecating

c) retain the suppository for a maximum of 5 minutes

d) expel the suppository immediately

A suppository prescribed for constipation is designed to soften the impacted faeces and thus aid defecation; the longer the patient can retain it the better. Some suppositories should be moistened with water before use; always read the manufacturer's instructions before use. The suppository should be gently introduced into the rectum and retained for at least 20 minutes to allow the chemicals to stimulate defecation.

19   **A specimen of urine from a patient with a urinary catheter should be:**

a) obtained from the urinary bag by draining urine from the exit port

b)   *obtained from the sampling ports using an aseptic technique*

c) obtained from any part of the catheter

d) obtained by removing the catheter and requesting the patient to void into a sterile dish

You must adhere to the principles of infection control when obtaining a catheter specimen of urine (CSU). The patient must be provided with sufficient information to provide consent, and dignity and privacy must be observed at all times. The specimen portal is cleaned using a recognized cleaning fluid (e.g. alcohol swab) and allowed to dry. A sterile needle is then inserted into the portal and a specimen of approximately 20 millilitres is withdrawn into the syringe. The specimen should be put into a sterile bottle specific for a CSU and the relevant bacteriology laboratory form completed before the specimen is sent to the laboratory.

20   **The urinary catheter balloon should be inflated using:**

a) air   b) tap water   *c) sterile water*   d) 0.9% sodium chloride

Sterile water is used to inflate the catheter balloon. The balloons come in various sizes; 10 millilitres of sterile water is normally recommended for adults. Catheterization is a sterile procedure and requires an aseptic technique.

21   **Presence of blood in the urine is defined as:**

a) haematemesis   b) haemoptysis   *c) haematuria*   d) haematocrit

The presence of blood in the urine is an indicator of infection, trauma to the urinary system, a disorder of the genito-urinary tract or an indicator of excess anticoagulant medication. Haematuria should always be investigated as it is also a feature of renal disease, thus further tests may be required to confirm a diagnosis.

22 **When collecting a catheter specimen of urine (CSU), if there is no urine present in the catheter tubing:**

a) clamp the catheter to allow urine to collect

b) take a sample from the catheter bag

c) *clamp the tubing below the sample port until sufficient urine collects*

d) disconnect the catheter to collect the specimen

If there is no urine present in the catheter tubing, clamp the tubing below the sample port until sufficient urine collects. Never clamp the catheter, as it could become damaged; and never disconnect the catheter, as this allows for the potential for infection. Always remember to unclamp the catheter after the specimen has been collected.

FILL IN THE BLANKS

23 **Catheterizing patients places them in significant danger of acquiring a _urinary tract infection_.**

Urinary tract infections (UTIs) are one of the most common bacterial infections treated in hospital. Infections of the urinary tract range from asymptomatic infections to severe sepsis, affecting high-risk patients such as diabetics or those receiving immunosuppressive therapy. Symptoms include frequency, dysuria and cystitis.

24 **Urine is normally _acidic_.**

Typical urine is normally yellow due to the pigment urochrome and slightly acidic (pH 6.0), but the pH can change as a result of dietary intake or metabolic processes. For example, a diet rich in meat tends to lead to acid production due to the chemical structure of the animal proteins. This will result in more acidic urine compared with vegetarians who will have a more alkaline urine.

25 **An indwelling catheter used in conjunction with an attached collection bag is known as a _closed circuit_.**

The closed circuit describes an indwelling catheter that is attached to a collection bag and is essentially closed to the exterior environment, thus limiting the number of entry routes for bacteria.

26 **Acute diarrhoea is usually caused by _bacteria_ and/or _viruses_.**

Antibacterial drugs are generally unnecessary in simple gastro-enteritis because the condition is usually associated with food and normally resolves without them. Infective diarrhoea that has a viral cause does not respond to antibiotics and again generally resolves spontaneously.

The priority for the nurse is to manage the associated symptoms and to prevent complications.

27 | **Increasing dietary *fibre* increases stool *bulk*, which in turn improves *peristalsis* and stool transit time.**

Peristalsis describes involuntary muscular contraction of the large bowel. The contraction constricts the bowel wall and squeezes the faecal material towards the rectum. This action is enhanced when there is adequate fibre in the diet. The fibre, particularly insoluble fibre such as that found in fruit and vegetable skins and wheat bran, increases stool bulk and speeds up the passage of faecal material through the bowel.

28 | **Individuals who suffer from constipation should be encouraged to increase their amount of *exercise*.**

Exercise, particularly aerobic exercise, increases the blood to muscles and therefore increases their ability to contract. This is known to have a positive effect on the peristalsis of the large bowel. Individuals who suffer from constipation should be encouraged to increase the amount of insoluble fibre in their diet and increase daily exercise.

29 | **The primary causes of constipation are inadequate diet, poor *fluid* intake, lifestyle change, ignoring the urge to *defecate*.**

Poor fluid intake can increase the risk of constipation due to inadequate amounts of fluid to make the bowel content soft. If the urge to defecate is ignored, the faeces remain in the colon for a longer period of time and there is excessive water absorption and the faeces become dry and hard.

30 | **Enemas are contraindicated in *paralytic ileus* and *colonic obstruction*.**

Paralytic ileus describes paralysis of the intestinal muscle and colonic obstruction describes a condition in which the bowel is obstructed. Both conditions are considered as medical emergencies and must be fully investigated before any attempt is made to evacuate the bowel. Any attempt to give an enema when these conditions are present could result in exacerbation of the condition and possible perforation of the bowel.

31 | **Stimulant laxatives increase intestinal *motility* by direct action on the *mucosa*.**

Stimulant laxatives increase intestinal motility and often cause abdominal cramp. They stimulate gastric emptying and small intestinal transit. Prolonged use of stimulant laxatives can cause diarrhoea and related effects from electrolyte imbalance.

32 **Correct sequence for doing a urinalysis using a reagent strip.**

1	Explain the procedure to the patient
2	Wash and dry hands and put on gloves and apron
3	Obtain a specimen of fresh urine from the patient
4	Check that the reagent sticks are in date
5	Dip the reagent stick into the urine. The strip should be completely immersed and then removed. Tap edge of strip gently along the container to remove excess urine
6	Hold the reagent stick at an angle
7	Wait the required time interval before reading the strip agent against the chart on the bottle
8	Dispose of urine sample in either the sluice or toilet
9	Remove apron and gloves and wash and dry hands
10	Document urinalysis reading and inform nurse in charge and medical staff of any abnormalities

6 Respiratory skills

INTRODUCTION

An efficient and healthy respiratory system is necessary to supply the cells and tissues of the body with oxygen and for the removal of carbon dioxide from the bloodstream. A decline in or absence of respiratory function represents a threat to health and well-being, as well as the continuation of life. It is, therefore, very important for nurses to develop skills and knowledge that will help them to assess and detect changes in respiratory function, often an early sign of potentially life-threatening deterioration in a person's condition, and to make appropriate nursing responses.

A change in normal respiratory function may occur due to the development of chronic diseases such as chronic obstructive pulmonary disease (COPD); alternatively, respiratory function may change rapidly due to acute exacerbation of a chronic respiratory illness (possibly due to infection). A change in respiratory function may also occur very rapidly, due to the effects of drugs (possibly anaesthetic drugs or opioids).

It is, therefore, essential for nurses to be able to assess and continuously monitor a person's respiratory function, and respond rapidly (in emergency situations) as well as to deliver appropriate nursing interventions when changes in function are detected. The ability to carry out a nursing assessment of the activity of breathing, diagnose problems amenable to nursing intervention and respond appropriately are essential skills.

Useful resources

Asthma UK:
http://www.asthma.org.uk/health_professionals/index.html

Nursing Times:
http://www.nursingtimes.net/section2.aspx?navcode=1335

Nurses! Test Yourself in Pathophysiology
Chapter 8

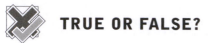

TRUE OR FALSE?

Are the following statements true or false?

1 Dyspnoea refers only to difficulty breathing in.

2 Normal respiration should be relatively silent.

3 Normal respiratory rate for an adult is 20–25 breaths per minute.

4 Breathlessness is *not* among the issues a nurse should ask about when assessing a patient with anaemia.

5 The administration of oxygen therapy to patients who have a chronically high partial pressure of arterial carbon dioxide ($PaCO_2$) – for example, those with COPD – is the first intervention of choice and should be continued until breathlessness improves.

6 Respiratory function may be influenced by a combination of age, environment, lifestyle, general health status, medications and stress.

7 Normal respiration requires patent airways, movement of air into and out of the lungs, gaseous exchange in the lungs and the transport of O_2 to and CO_2 from body tissues.

8 The oropharyngeal airway should be used only in patients with impaired consciousness due to recent general anaesthesia, overdose or brain injury.

9 Many patients who require suctioning have respiratory disease and suctioning can induce hypoxia in some of these patients.

10 The water level, in a water-sealed chest drain, should remain constant during inspiration and expiration.

MULTIPLE CHOICE

Identify one correct answer for each of the following.

11 Nasal (nostril) flaring and lip pursing may indicate:

a) respiratory tract infection

b) anxiety

c) respiratory distress

d) shock

12 Which of the following oxygen delivery systems delivers a low concentration of oxygen?

a) partial rebreather mask

b) nasal cannula (nasal specs)

c) simple face mask

d) Venturi mask

13 In the delivery of nebulizer therapy, the O_2 flow meter should be set so that a fine mist is delivered from the face mask. This is normally achieved at a rate of:

a) 2–4 litres per minute

b) 4–6 litres per minute

c) 6–8 litres per minute

d) 8–10 litres per minute

14 Which of the following is an advantage of dry powder inhalers that should be considered by nurses?

a) they are lighter than other types of inhaler

b) they are more effective than metered dose inhalers because the powder is absorbed more easily

c) they are more hygienic than other types of inhalers

d) they do not require coordination of inhalation with manual activation of the device

15 In teaching how to use a pressured metered dose inhaler (pMDI), which of the following should a nurse impress upon a patient, *following inspiration*?

a) hold breath for 10 seconds, or as long as possible, then breathe out slowly

b) hold breath for 20 seconds, or as long as possible, then breathe out slowly

c) following inhalation of the medication, holding breath is not important; breathe normally

d) holding breath is important only for people with COPD

16 Humidification of O_2 is *not* required:

a) in long-term use

b) in home situations

c) in patients who do not have excessive secretions

d) in low flow O_2 delivery systems, such as with a nasal cannula

17 Spirometry is contraindicated in patients with:

a) COPD

b) asthma

c) bronchiectasis

d) recent thoracic, eye or abdominal surgery

18 Which of the following are *not* signs of deterioration in a patient with asthma?

a) cannot complete a sentence due to breathlessness

b) peak expiratory flow <40% of predicted or best attained <200 litres per minute

c) respiratory rate is persistently >25 breaths per minute and pulse is persistently >110 beats per minute

d) elevated body temperature

FILL IN THE BLANKS

Fill in the blanks in each statement using the words in the box below.
Not all of them are required, so choose carefully.

spacer device	chronic obstructive pulmonary disease
hypoxaemia	respiratory rate and depth
pulmonary embolism	stop
orthopnoea	deep venous thrombosis
suctioning	hypoxia
pursed lip breathing	inhaler device

19 _____ is a difficulty in breathing when lying down.

20 When administering certain types of medication, a nurse must pay particular attention to the _____.

21 _____ may be deemed necessary by the presence of noises associated with inspiration and expiration.

22 A _____ is a large plastic (or metal) container with a mouthpiece at one end and an opening to fit an inhaler to at the other.

23 Nurses, and other prescribers, should ensure that an _____ is matched to an individual patient's needs and abilities.

24 An estimated 3 million people have _____ in the UK.

25 _____ refers to low levels of O_2 in the cells.

26 Sudden onset of acute breathlessness, along with chest pain and distress, may be an indication of _____.

27 Nurses who work in primary/community care or in hospitals should advise everyone who smokes to _____.

28 When a patient has an ineffective breathing pattern related to dyspnoea, this may be helped by teaching _____.

LABELLING EXERCISE

29–36 Identify the types of inhaler in Figure 6.1, using the names provided in the box below:

Accuhaler   Diskhaler

Easi-Breathe   Autohaler

Metered dose inhaler   Spinhaler

Spacer device   Turbohaler

Figure 6.1 Types of inhaler

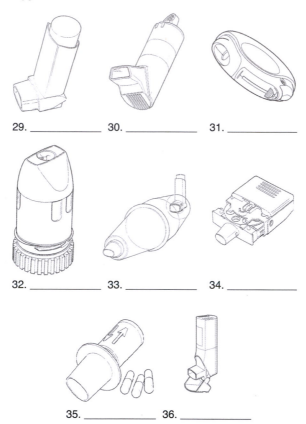

29. _____ 30. _____ 31. _____

32. _____ 33. _____ 34. _____

35. _____ 36. _____

ANSWERS

TRUE OR FALSE?

1 | **Dyspnoea refers only to difficulty breathing in.**

Dyspnoea refers to any undue awareness of difficulty breathing in or out. In assessing a patient, you should ask about any perceived problem with breathing; you should also notice if the person is 'dyspnoeic on exertion'. If a person reports (or shows) signs of having difficulty breathing on movement, you should try to quantify how much movement induces breathlessness (walking up stairs, or walking ten paces on the level). Your assessment may also reveal a person to be 'dyspnoeic at rest'; this will become evident if the person reports (or shows) signs of difficulty breathing while inactive (sitting or lying).

2 | **Normal respiration should be relatively silent.**

When assessing a person's breathing, it is important to listen. In normal breathing, there should not be any obvious sounds associated with inspiration or expiration. Normal, relaxed breathing should be effortless, automatic, regular and almost silent. If wheezing or coughing are present, this is abnormal and should be noted.

3 | **Normal respiratory rate for an adult is 20–25 breaths per minute.**

Normal respiratory rate for an adult ranges from 12 to 20 breaths per minute with an average of 16 breaths per minute being usual. When assessing a person, any substantial deviation from this range may be clinically significant and should be noted. Rapid breathing, in excess of 20 breaths per minute, is clinically significant and must be monitored vigilantly. Should assessment reveal a respiratory rate substantially below 10 breaths per minute, this requires prompt action and may be the prelude to a catastrophic deterioration in a person's health.

4 | **Breathlessness is *not* among the issues a nurse should ask about when assessing a patient with anaemia.**

A nurse should be aware that anaemia causes reduced oxygen-carrying capacity, due to lower levels of haemoglobin. This can lead to an anaemic patient experiencing feelings of breathlessness and having abnormally low oxygen saturation levels; this would be a potentially serious omission on respiratory assessment.

5 | **The administration of oxygen therapy to patients who have a chronically high partial pressure of arterial carbon dioxide ($PaCO_2$) – for example, those with COPD – is the first intervention of choice and should be continued until breathlessness improves.** ✖

People with a chronically elevated $PaCO_2$ are stimulated to breathe by low levels of oxygen, also known as the hypoxic drive. Therefore, the administration of high concentrations of oxygen may raise the O_2 level and, consequently, remove the stimulus to breathe, possibly resulting in respiratory depression. Oxygen should be considered a drug and should be administered only in response to careful assessment of an individual's condition and usually following medical prescription.

6 | **Respiratory function may be influenced by a combination of age, environment, lifestyle, general health status, medications and stress.** ✔

When assessing and delivering care to a patient, a nurse must take account of the possible part played by various issues in relation to breathing: lifestyle choices (smoking), underlying health conditions (heart disease, respiratory disease), medications (opioid analgesia), as well as the possible effect of employment and even city living. These aspects of a person's history may be clinically relevant in respiratory assessment.

7 | **Normal respiration requires patent airways, movement of air into and out of the lungs, gaseous exchange in the lungs and the transport of O_2 to and CO_2 from body tissues.** ✔

When assessing the respiratory function of a patient, a nurse must consider all of the above. Conditions that cause spasm or narrowing of the air passages, over-production of sputum, cardiac arrest where a patient is not breathing, bronchial oedema (in which alveoli are not available for gaseous exchange), heart failure or hypovolaemia can all produce changes in respiratory function. Nurses must be able to identify the specific respiratory changes and then understand the possible underlying causes.

8 | **The oropharyngeal airway should be used only in patients with impaired consciousness due to recent general anaesthesia, overdose or brain injury.** ✔

The oropharyngeal airway should be used only in patients who have had recent general anaesthetic and who are not fully alert, those who have impaired consciousness through overdose or have drowsiness due to recent head injury. It protects the upper air passage from becoming compromised by the tongue and it stimulates the gag reflex when a patient becomes adequately alert and conscious.

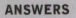

9 | **Many patients who require suctioning have respiratory disease and suctioning can induce hypoxia in some of these patients.** ✓

Poorly executed suctioning that takes too long, or is carried out by an inexperienced nurse, who does not observe the patient closely during the procedure, may result in a distressed and hypoxic patient. The procedure may induce prolonged coughing and interfere with the established breathing pattern; it may also increase discomfort and anxiety, thus interfering with breathing. Each passage of suctioning should last no more than 10 seconds and time should be allowed for the patient to recover. The nurse should also closely observe the patient during the procedure for signs of distress. The procedure should be stopped if this becomes apparent.

10 | **The water level, in a water-sealed chest drain, should remain constant during inspiration and expiration.** ✗

A water-sealed drain is designed to drain fluid or air from the chest cavity via a drain. This is commonly inserted to allow for the re-inflation of a collapsed lung. However, it is very important that, when air leaves the chest cavity, none is allowed to re-enter the cavity. Therefore, a system must be in place that allows air to leave freely, but in such a manner that it cannot re-enter. This is achieved by placing the end of the drainage tube under water (underwater sealed drain). Air can leave via the drain, enter the water and bubble away, but further air cannot re-enter because the end of the drain is under water. It is very important for a nurse to observe that the level of water in the seal is rising and falling (sometimes called swinging) in relation to the chest pressure changes associated with inspiration and expiration.

MULTIPLE CHOICE

Correct answers identified in bold italics

11 | **Nasal (nostril) flaring and lip pursing may indicate:**

a) respiratory tract infection   b) anxiety   *c) respiratory distress*
d) shock

In an adult with a healthy respiratory tract, normal breathing should be almost imperceptible. The intercostal muscles and the diaphragm are, normally, the only muscles needed to assist in breathing. However, when a patient is in respiratory distress, much greater effort is expended and other muscle groups are needed to assist with breathing; these 'accessory' muscles include the trapezius, sternomastoids and the scalenes. Normal breathing does not usually involve the muscles of the face. However, in respiratory distress, a nurse may also see 'nasal flaring', an attempt to widen the entry to the nasal passages; this is not usual and should be seen by the nurse as clinically significant.

12 **Which of the following oxygen delivery systems delivers a low concentration of oxygen?:**

a) partial rebreather mask   *b) nasal cannula (nasal specs)*
c) simple face mask   d) Venturi mask

Oxygen should be considered a drug and, with the possible exception of emergencies, should be administered on medical prescription only. The concentration (dose) of O_2 required depends on the condition being treated. Nurses must know that, wrongly used, O_2 has the potential to have serious or even fatal consequences. A nurse might expect to see high concentrations of O_2 being used in cases of pneumonia, sepsis, shock or severe trauma. However, there are conditions in which this might be dangerous; accordingly, lower concentrations of O_2 are required, for example, in those with COPD or where respiratory depression due to opioid overdose is a risk. Administering O_2 via a nasal cannula means the O_2 is not being concentrated. From a nursing point of view, a nasal cannula allows the patient to talk, eat and drink; however, nasal mucosa can become dry and painful. It is a nurse's responsibility to be knowledgeable about O_2 delivery systems and to appreciate the possible dangers associated with delivering O_2 in the wrong concentrations by using the wrong delivery system. Nurses might usefully consult an up-to-date British National Formulary and read the section about oxygen use.

13 **In the delivery of nebulizer therapy, the O_2 flow meter should be set so that a fine mist is delivered from the face mask. This is normally achieved at a rate of:**

a) 2–4 litres per minute   b) 4–6 litres per minute
c) 6–8 litres per minute   d) 8–10 litres per minute

A nebulizer converts a solution of drug into an aerosol for inhalation into the lungs. A range of drugs can be delivered in this way, including corticosteroids, bronchodilators and antibiotics. If a diluent is needed, it is normally saline 0.9%. Nurses should remember that they are administering a drug, so the normal protocols about legal prescriptions and checking procedures (drug and patient identity) must be applied. The nebulizing effect is achieved by setting the O_2 flow rate to between 6 and 8 litres per minute, producing a fine mist from the mask. The nurse should leave the nebulizer in place until all of the drug has been delivered. The patient should be made comfortable and encouraged to breathe normally while the nebulizer is in place. Afterwards, the patient may feel the need to cough, so the nurse should ensure tissues and a sputum carton are within reach.

14 **Which of the following is an advantage of dry powder inhalers that should be considered by nurses?**

a) they are lighter than other types of inhaler

b) they are more effective than metered dose inhalers because the powder is absorbed more easily

c) they are more hygienic than other types of inhalers

d) *they do not require coordination of inhalation with manual activation of the device*

Selecting an inhaler to suit an individual patient's needs is very important; if a device is not being used properly, the prescribed drug may not be being delivered deep into the respiratory tract, which can lead to more frequent exacerbations of the illness, more hospital admissions and poorer quality of life for the patient. Therefore, nurses must ensure that inhaler devices are matched to a patient's particular needs and abilities. Some patients may be unable to inhale efficiently enough for breath-activated inhalers, while some may struggle with the dexterity and coordination required manually to activate pressured metered dose inhalers at precisely the right point. With dry powder inhalers (DPIs), the patient does not have to coordinate inhalation with activating the inhaler. A potential problem that nurses should address with the patient is that some DPIs need to be loaded and patients with poor hand strength or coordination may struggle with this. The nurse should demonstrate this loading process and assess whether or not the patient can do it.

15 **In teaching how to use a pressured metered dose inhaler (pMDI), which of the following should a nurse impress upon a patient, *following inspiration*?**

a) *hold breath for 10 seconds, or as long as possible, then breathe out slowly*

b) hold breath for 20 seconds, or as long as possible, then breathe out slowly

c) following inhalation of the medication, holding breath is not important; breathe normally

d) holding breath is important only for people with COPD

In teaching a patient to use a pMDI, a nurse should ask the patient to remove the cap and shake the inhaler. The patient should breathe out gently, then place the mouthpiece in the mouth. At the start of a slow, deep inspiration, the canister should be pressed down; the patient should continue to breathe in deeply *through the mouth*. At this point, the patient should be asked to hold their breath for 10 seconds, or as long as able, and then breathe out slowly. Some patients may struggle to coordinate pressing the canister precisely with breathing in; they may press too soon or too late and the drug may be seen to escape into the atmosphere in front of the patient's face, meaning the drug has not been administered, and no therapeutic effect is gained.

16 Humidification of O_2 is *not* required:

a) in long-term use

b) in home situations

c) in patients who do not have excessive secretions

d) *in low flow O_2 delivery systems, such as with a nasal cannula*

Humidification is the amount of water present in the environment. Inspired atmospheric air contains varying percentages of water, depending on prevailing conditions. Air travelling through the air passages is warmed, moistened and filtered before it reached the lungs. Normally, by the time air reaches the alveoli, it is fully humidified and warmed to around 37°C. This process can be impaired through disease or dehydration. Should this happen, the nurse must take measures to humidify air entering the respiratory tract. Should a nurse fail to consider this, further drying of the mucous membranes will take place along with drying of pulmonary secretions, making it very difficult for a patient to cough these secretions from his or her respiratory tract. The O_2 is passed through water on its way to the patient and a water vapour is produced (often 20–40% humidity), which moistens the air passages, thus helping protect the mucosa and also helping moisten and loosen pulmonary secretions. However, when O_2 is being delivered via low flow systems (1–2 litres per minute), such as a nasal cannula, humidification is not usually required because sufficient room air is usually inhaled along with the O_2 being delivered via the nasal cannula.

17 Spirometry is contraindicated in patients with:

a) COPD   b) asthma   c) bronchiectasis

d) *recent thoracic, eye or abdominal surgery*

Spirometry measures the flow of air inhaled or exhaled through a mouthpiece. This procedure can be carried out by appropriately trained staff in hospital or in primary care settings. It is used to help investigate respiratory symptoms (dyspnoea, wheeze, cough), and its use should be considered in people who have regular chest infections. Specialist nurses also use it to monitor established respiratory disease such as asthma or COPD or to diagnose new cases. The nurse should advise a patient not to wear restrictive clothing when having the test and not to eat a large meal in the two hours beforehand. He should not drink alcohol before the test and should try not to smoke in the 24 hours before testing. He should also be advised not to exercise vigorously prior to the test (although for many people with established disease, this advice may not be necessary). While there are no absolute contraindications to the use of spirometry, the nurse should proceed with caution in the following circumstances:

- known/suspected respiratory infection
- haemoptysis of unknown origin
- unstable cardiovascular problems such as recent myocardial infarction or hypertension
- history of haemorrhagic stroke
- recent thoracic, eye or abdominal surgery

18 | **Which of the following are *not* signs of deterioration in a patient with asthma?**

a) cannot complete a sentence due to breathlessness

b) peak expiratory flow <40% of predicted or best attained <200 litres per minute

c) respiratory rate is persistently >25 breaths per minute and pulse persistently >110 beats per minute

d) *elevated body temperature*

Asthma carries a mortality rate and acute flare-ups can become life-threatening in some patients. Therefore, a nurse needs to closely monitor the patient's condition and develop skills in assessing improvement or deterioration in the condition of someone having an asthma attack. If a patient begins to become so breathless that he cannot complete a short sentence due to breathlessness, this must be noted as a possible sign of deterioration. Measurement of peak expiratory flow (PEF) can be a useful means by which to monitor the effectiveness of treatment or possible improvement; however, if it becomes apparent that the patient can blow only about 40% of previously best attained rate, then the nurse must consider this as a point of danger and have the patient's condition medically reviewed. A persistent heart rate of more than 110 beats per minute together with tachypnoea above 25 breaths per minute indicates a degree of distress that requires medical assessment. A nurse should be aware that a patient with any combination of these signs may deteriorate very rapidly, so prompt action is necessary. Should the nurse fail to recognize these signs as serious, a patient may begin to show signs of imminent threat to life, such as cyanosis, bradycardia (not to be mistaken for improvement), no chest sounds on auscultation and exhaustion, confusion or unconsciousness. An elevated body temperature in someone with an asthma flare-up, while it should be dealt with, is not unusual.

FILL IN THE BLANKS

19 *Orthopnoea* **is a difficulty in breathing when lying down.**

Orthopnoea is usually relieved when the patient is assisted into an upright position. It is an important observation to be made on respiratory assessment and is often associated with left ventricular failure (LVF) and pulmonary oedema. Several things make breathing less efficient when a person is lying flat; greater blood volume in the thoracic cavity and compression of the chest. This, when combined in a patient who has LVF and pulmonary oedema, means that the alveoli are filled with fluid and are therefore not available for gaseous exchange. Nursing a patient in the orthopnoeic position will, therefore, reduce the volume of blood in the chest and decrease the level of fluid in the alveoli, thus making the alveoli available again for gaseous exchange and improving breathing.

20 **When administering certain types of medication, a nurse must pay particular attention to the** *respiratory rate and depth.*

Some medication can cause changes to breathing; this is especially important when administered for the first time or when the dosage is increased. Nurses must be especially vigilant when administering opioid analgesia, which can cause respiratory depression. Similar issues need to be considered with patients who have taken an overdose of benzodiazepine drugs.

21 *Suctioning* **may be deemed necessary by the presence of noises associated with inspiration and expiration.**

When a patient is unable to remove his own secretions from the respiratory tract (because they are too copious, too viscous, disease has narrowed the air passages or because he is too exhausted to cough), and this situation is allowed to continue without intervention, then some more problems may become apparent. Changes in the rate and pattern of respiration, increased restlessness, anxiety and decreased O_2 saturation are all things a nurse should include in her observation schedule when caring for a patient who has a respiratory illness; suctioning may be necessary to help a patient clear secretions.

22 **A** *spacer device* **is a large plastic (or metal) container with a mouthpiece at one end and an opening to fit an inhaler to at the other.**

A spacer can be used with a pressured metered dose inhaler (pMDI) only and a nurse should consider its use when a patient cannot successfully coordinate manual activation of a pMDI with inspiration, thus allowing the drug to escape into the air.

23 | **Nurses, and other prescribers, should ensure that an *inhaler device* is matched to an individual patient's needs and abilities.**

Inhalers, properly used, represent an efficient method of delivering drugs directly into the respiratory tract. The drugs can be delivered in powder form or in aerosol form. Inhalers can be breath-activated or manually activated. Dry powder inhalers are breath-activated (the act of breathing in through the mouth via the inhaler delivers the drug). This means that the patient does not have to coordinate manual activation, by pressing a canister, with breathing in. However, a nurse should check if the patient can breathe in vigorously enough to activate the inhaler; some powder inhalers need to be loaded or primed and this may be difficult for some patients. Alternatively, some pMDIs can be breath-activated; a nurse should also consider if the patient is capable of activating these inhalers by breathing in. Some pMDIs need to be manually activated. However, they may not be suitable for patients with poor coordination or arthritis and they may be unsuitable for children. Spacer devices can be used with pMDIs to help solve some of these problems but the canister still needs to be used, so spacers may not help people with poor hand strength, such as those with arthritis.

24 | **An estimated 3 million people have *chronic obstructive pulmonary disease* in the UK.**

Nurses should have an understanding of the prevalence of respiratory disease in the population. Most people are not diagnosed with COPD until they are in their fifties. It is predominantly caused by smoking and results in airflow obstruction that is not normally reversible. Nurses working in hospital or non-hospital environments should consider the possibility of COPD in any smoker over the age of 35, who presents with exertional breathlessness, chronic cough, regular sputum production and frequent winter wheeze or chest infection. The condition does not normally get worse over months but, in the longer term, it is progressive. Nurses will see patients with acute deterioration in their condition and a worsening in the severity of their symptoms beyond their normal state, especially during winter months. Aside from the nursing role of caring for people with established disease, nurses may have a role in prevention of this condition by taking opportunities to encourage people to make healthier lifestyle choices, particularly in relation to smoking behaviour.

25 | **_Hypoxia_ refers to low levels of O_2 in the cells.**

Hypoxaemia refers to low levels of O_2 in the bloodstream; this may be caused by anything that interferes with gaseous exchange in the alveoli (atelectasis or pulmonary oedema). The nurse should also be alert to the fact that hypoxaemia may also be caused by anaemia due to insufficient oxygen-carrying capacity of the red cells. A nurse should be aware of how the cardiovascular system may try to compensate for this condition by an increase in heart rate and cardiac output. Correct interpretation of these signs by the nurse is very important. If this condition is not recognized and reversed, hypoxia will ensue, a low level of O_2 in the cells. The nurse should recognize this as a further deterioration that may be identified by an increase in pulse rate, rapid, shallow respirations, dyspnoea, restlessness, agitation, sometimes confusion, and rapidly developing cyanosis. Inspection of the oral mucosa by the nurse will reveal a bluish tinge, indicating central cyanosis and tissue hypoxia. The nurse must be alert to this rapidly developing situation and secure urgent medical assessment and treatment.

26 **Sudden onset of acute breathlessness, along with chest pain and distress, may be an indication of *pulmonary embolism.***

Formation of a thrombus in the venous system may be dangerous for the patient; however, a small portion of the thrombus may break away (embolus) and travel rapidly until it becomes lodged in the small blood vessels in the lungs, where it is termed a 'pulmonary embolism'. Sudden, unexpected difficulty breathing along with chest pain may be the first indication to the nurse that something has happened. Oxygen saturation, when checked, may be lower than might normally be expected. This may be accompanied by cyanosis, tachycardia, cough or haemoptysis. A nurse should recognize these symptoms immediately and set in train rapid medical assessment and treatment.

27 **Nurses who work in primary/community care or in hospitals should advise everyone who smokes to *stop.***

Given the strong link between smoking and respiratory disease, nurses may have a role to play in helping those who smoke to stop. Nurses might usefully refer to the N I C E recommendations in relation to the use of brief interventions to assist people to consider stopping smoking. Everyone who smokes should be advised to stop. The nurse should investigate how interested a patient may be in stopping. Nurses should be familiar with the facilities in their areas or own N H S Trust to whom patients may be referred for counselling or pharmacotherapeutic support. Smoking cessation advice should be available to every smoker who comes into contact with any part of the health service and nurses should expect to play a unique role in this. Nurses should encourage smokers to consider stopping or refer them to the appropriate support services.

28 **When a patient has an ineffective breathing pattern related to dyspnoea, this may be helped by teaching *pursed lip breathing.***

Nurses should consider teaching patients with a breathing difficulty (related to obstructive respiratory diseases) specialized breathing techniques. One such technique is called pursed lip breathing. It can help a patient re-establish an effective cycle of inhaling and exhaling. It requires no equipment and can be carried out anywhere at any time. It can improve lung ventilation, and decrease the work of breathing. It prolongs the phase of expiration, slows the respiratory rate and makes breathing more efficient. The nurse should ask the patient to relax their neck and shoulder muscles. The patient should then be asked to breathe in slowly through the nose for a count of two; this should not be a deep breath, but something which the patient finds comfortable. The patient should then be asked to purse his lips (as if going to whistle) and breathe out slowly and gently; breathing out should be for a count of four (inhale on two, exhale on four). This technique should be practised by the patient; it helps regain control of breathing, establishes a slower, more efficient effective breathing pattern, and can also help with a more general mental state or relaxation.

LABELLING EXERCISE

Figure 6.2 Types of inhaler

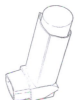
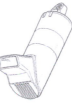

29. Metered dose inhaler   30. Accuhaler   31. Autohaler

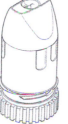

32. Turbohaler   33. Spacer device   34. Diskhaler

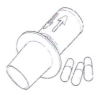

35. Spinhaler   36. Easi-Breathe

7 Cardiovascular skills

INTRODUCTION

This chapter introduces you to the skills required to assess a patient's cardiovascular status. To complete a proper assessment, it is not enough just to be able to do the skill. You will also need some knowledge of the theory underpinning your practice. You will also need to revise the basic anatomy and physiology associated with the cardiovascular system. It is important that you learn skills and knowledge in tandem.

The cardiovascular system has benefited from advances in surgical, medical and pharmacological advances over the years. As a nurse, you will be responsible for much of the care delivered and it is vital that you have an understanding of, and are competent in, the skills associated with cardiovascular nursing.

Useful resources

Mader's Understanding Human Anatomy and Physiology

Nurses! Test Yourself in Pathophysiology
Chapter 7

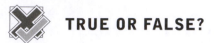 **TRUE OR FALSE?**

Are the following statements true or false?

1 The pulse is a good indicator of the heart rate.

2 The respiratory rate is inconsequential to the patient's overall well-being.

3 The degree of oxygenation affects skin colour.

4 The normal value for capillary refill time (CRT) is <2 seconds.

5 The standard approach when assessing the deteriorating or ill patient is ABCDE.

6 Blood pressure refers to the pressure blood exerts on the vessel in which it is contained.

7 Before recording blood pressure, it is important to estimate the systolic pressure by inflating the cuff until the radial pulse can no longer be felt.

8 Taking a pulse for <60 seconds is appropriate.

MULTIPLE CHOICE

Identify one correct answer for each of the following.

9 When measuring manual blood pressure, the cuff of the sphygmomanometer should be placed over:

a) the brachial artery

b) the radial artery

c) the abdominal artery

d) the carotid artery

10 Bradycardia is used to describe a heart rate that is:

a) irregular

b) weak and thready

c) pulsating and >60 beats per minute

d) slow and <60 beats per minute

11 When measuring blood pressure, it is important to:

a) select the correct cuff size

b) palpate the carotid artery

c) inflate 50–60 mmHg above where you cannot feel sensation in either the brachial or radial artery

d) remember that the first Korotkoff sound is the diastolic pressure

12 Tachycardia is used to describe a heart rate that is:

a) irregular

b) weak and thready

c) pulsating and >100 beats per minute

d) slow and <60 beats per minute

13 Cardiac enzymes are found in:

a) cholesterol

b) soft tissue

c) subcutaneous tissue

d) cardiac tissue

14 Pulse oximetry estimates:

a) arterial oxygen saturation

b) arterial carbon dioxide saturation

c) arterial nitrogen saturation

d) venous oxygen saturation

15 Patients presenting with chest pain should always have:

a) an EEG

b) an Echo

c) an ECG

d) an ERCP

16 Phlebitis in the lower calf region of the leg can indicate:

a) infection

b) drug allergy

c) fracture

d) deep venous thrombosis

17 Patients most at risk of developing a deep venous thrombosis are:

a) post-operative patients

b) ambulatory patients

c) pre-operative patients

d) asthmatic patients

FILL IN THE BLANKS

Fill in the blanks in each statement using the words in the box below.
Not all of them are required, so choose carefully.

arteries	oxygen
Korotkoff	brachial
radial	80%
carbon dioxide	CPR
160 mmHg	pulsate
sternum	chin
100 mmHg	abdomen
head	neck
feel	veins

18 The systolic blood pressure provides information about the status of the heart and great _____.

19 Blood pressure measurements are recorded in association with _____ sounds.

20 When measuring blood pressure, the cuff should be inflated until the _____ pulse can no longer be felt.

21 When measuring blood pressure, it is important to use a cuff that covers _____ of the circumference of the upper arm.

22 The British Hypertension Society recommends that patients who have sustained systolic blood pressure of greater than or equal to _____, or sustained diastolic blood pressure of greater or equal to _____, should be commenced on anti-hypertensive drug treatment.

23 When a patient has no signs of life, no pulse, or if there is any doubt, start _____ immediately.

24 The correct hand position for chest compression is in the middle of the lower half of the _____.

25 In the case of a collapsed patient who is unresponsive, the patient should be turned on his back and the airway opened using the _____ tilt and _____ lift.

26 Airway assessment should be performed using the look, listen and _____ approach.

ANSWERS

TRUE OR FALSE?

1 | **The pulse is a good indicator of the heart rate.** ✔

The arterial pulse is one of the measurements used to assess the condition of the heart. Each time the heart beats, it pushes blood into the aorta and then through the peripheral arteries. The pumping action of the heart causes the walls of the arteries to expand and distend, causing a wave-like sensation which can be felt as the pulse.

2 | **The respiratory rate is inconsequential to the patient's overall well-being.** ✖

The respiratory rate is the primary indicator of a patient's overall well-being. Changes to the patient's cardiovascular system and neurological system will manifest as an altered respiratory rate. The respiratory centre, located in the medulla oblongata in the brain, is responsible for breathing.

3 | **The degree of oxygenation affects skin colour.** ✔

The degree of oxygenation affects skin colour. Haemoglobin, attached to red blood cells, transports oxygen to the tissues. A diminished flow of oxyhaemoglobin through the cutaneous circulation results in pallor. In people with light skin, the skin appears very pale, without the usual pink undertones. In people with darker skin, pallor manifests as a yellowish-brown or ashen appearance (again, because the usual pink undertones are lost).

4 | **The normal value for capillary refill time (CRT) is <2 seconds.** ✔

Capillary refill time is measured by applying sufficient pressure on a fingertip or toe to cause blanching. The pressure is removed after 5 seconds and then it is timed how long it takes for the skin to return to the colour of the surrounding skin. The normal value for CRT is usually <2 seconds. A prolonged CRT suggests poor peripheral perfusion.

5 | **The standard approach when assessing the deteriorating or ill patient is ABCDE.** ✔

ABCDE refers to Airway, Breathing, Circulation, Disability and Exposure.

When using ABCDE, it is important to complete a full assessment and reassess regularly. It is important to recognize when you need help and to call for appropriate help early.

6 | **Blood pressure refers to the pressure blood exerts on the vessel in which it is contained.** ✓

Blood pressure is a normal physiological occurrence within the human body and is simply the pressure exerted on the blood vessels. However, there are times when the blood pressure can fall below what is considered normal (hypotension) and equally it can rise above what is considered to be normal (hypertension). Both hypotension and hypertension can have serious consequences. Blood pressure is usually expressed as millimetres of mercury (mmHg).

7 | **Before recording blood pressure, it is important to estimate the systolic pressure by inflating the cuff until the radial pulse can no longer be felt.** ✓

This serves two purposes. First, it reduces the margin for error in patients who have an auscultatory gap. An auscultatory gap is when Korotkoff sounds disappear shortly after the systolic pressure is heard and resume well above what corresponds to the diastolic pressure. Second, it removes the need to over-inflate the cuff and cause potential discomfort to the patient.

8 | **Taking a pulse for <60 seconds is appropriate.** ✗

The pulse should be counted for 60 seconds. This allows for sufficient time to detect any irregularities or other defects. Pulses can be described according to their characteristics. For example, pulsus alternans is a pulse that alternates in strength with every other beat; it is often found in patients with left ventricular failure. Pulsus paradoxus is a pulse that disappears during inspiration but returns during expiration.

MULTIPLE CHOICE

Correct answers identified in bold italics

9 | **When measuring manual blood pressure, the cuff of the sphygmomanometer should be placed over:**

a) the brachial artery   b) the radial artery   c) the abdominal artery
d) the carotid artery

Arterial blood pressure is the pressure of blood in the arteries and arterioles. It is a pulsatile pressure due to the cardiac cycle, and systolic and diastolic numbers are reported in millimetres of mercury. The brachial artery branches from the arch of the aorta via the subclavian and axillary arteries. It is the preferred artery to obtain a correct reading when taking a manual blood pressure.

10 **Bradycardia is used to describe a heart rate that is:**

a) irregular

b) weak and thready

c) pulsating and >60 beats per minute

d) slow and <60 beats per minute

Bradycardia is a heart rate slower than 60 beats per minute. It may be physiological, as in athletes when physical and cardiovascular conditioning occurs; it may be cardiac in origin, e.g. atrioventricular block or sinus node disease; it may be non-cardiac in origin, e.g. vasovagal, hypothermia, hypothyroidism, hyperkalaemia; or it may be drug-induced, e.g. beta blockers, digoxin, amiodarone.

11 **When measuring blood pressure, it is important to:**

a) select the correct cuff size

b) palpate the carotid artery

c) inflate 50–60 mmHg above where you cannot feel sensation in either the brachial or radial artery

d) remember that the first Korotkoff sound is the diastolic pressure

It is very important to select the correct cuff size. The cuff is normally made of washable material or is disposable. Velcro is usually used to secure it around the arm. Obese patients need large cuffs, children small ones. If you take blood pressure in an obese patient with a standard cuff, you will get a falsely high reading, as the cuff has to exert a greater pressure to compress the artery.

12 **Tachycardia is used to describe a heart rate that is:**

a) irregular

b) weak and thready

c) pulsating and >100 beats per minute

d) slow and <60 beats per minute

Tachycardia is defined as an abnormally fast heart rate, over 100 beats per minute in adults. It can occur as a result of a raised body temperature, increased sympathetic response due to physical/emotional stress, certain drugs or heart disease. When you feel the radial pulse and find it to be tachycardic, you should consider the rhythm – regular or irregular? If irregular, how does it vary? You may wish to recommend an ECG to confirm your findings. You should also feel the carotid pulse, as the character of the pulse is best assessed at the carotid artery.

13   Cardiac enzymes are found in:

a) cholesterol   b) soft tissue   c) subcutaneous tissue   *d) cardiac tissue*

Cardiac enzymes are found in cardiac tissue. When cardiac injury occurs as in acute myocardial infarction (MI), these enzymes are released into the serum, and their concentrations can be measured. Although cardiac damage does result in above-normal serum concentrations of these enzymes, the quantification of cardiac enzyme levels, along with other diagnostic tests and the clinical presentation of the patient, is routinely used for diagnosing cardiac disease, particularly acute MI.

14   Pulse oximetry estimates:

a) *arterial oxygen saturation*   b) arterial carbon dioxide saturation

c) arterial nitrogen saturation   d) venous oxygen saturation

Pulse oximetry estimates arterial oxygen saturation or the percentage of haemoglobin saturated with oxygen. Oxygen saturation and haemoglobin are the two major components of arterial oxygen content (CaO_2). If arterial oxygen content is decreased for any reason, cardiac output (mostly heart rate) increases to compensate. When a patient cannot increase cardiac output, as in heart failure, then even modest decreases in CaO_2 produce symptoms and increase the likelihood of an exacerbation or death. You should always be concerned about a patient with a pulse oximetry reading of <90%.

15   Patients presenting with chest pain should always have:

a) an EEG   b) an Echo   *c) an ECG*   d) an ERCP

The electrocardiogram (ECG) is used to assess rate and rhythm. An ECG should always be recorded when a patient presents with chest pain. It is useful in diagnosing arrhythmias, conduction defects and myocardial infarction. An ECG can also distinguish frequent permanent ventricular beats that are common in acute and chronic heart failure. The waveforms, which indicate the electrical activity of the myocardium, are analysed using the ECG tracing.

- *P wave* – represents atrial depolarization, indicating the contraction of both atria. The P wave is usually smooth and upright or 'positive'.

- *PR interval* – is measured from the beginning of the P wave (onset of atrial depolarization) to the R wave. It represents the time required for atrial depolarization and for the impulse to travel through the entire conduction system and Purkinje fibre network. A normal PR interval is 0.12 to 0.20 seconds.

- *QRS complex* – represents depolarization of the ventricles, which causes the ventricular contraction.

- *ST segment* – represents the period of early ventricular repolarization. The ST segment is normally isoelectric (line is flat).

■   *QT interval* – represents the total time required for ventricular depolarization and repolarization.

■   *T wave* – represents ventricular repolarization or the return of the ventricles to a resting state.

16 **Phlebitis in the lower calf region of the leg can indicate:**

a) infection   b) drug allergy   c) fracture   *d) deep venous thrombosis*

Most hospitalized patients have multiple risk factors for developing deep vein thrombosis. Primary factors include hypercoagulable state, venous stasis and vascular (endothelial) injury. These factors lead to platelet aggregation, fibrin, WBC and RBC deposition, and eventual formation of a free-floating clot. In 80% of cases, clots begin in the deep veins of the calf. Within 7–10 days, the clot adheres to the vein wall, phelibitis develops, the clot is invaded by fibroblasts, scar is formed and blood is restored, but the vein valves are usually permanently damaged. The clot propagates proximally; pieces can break off and embolize to the heart and obstruct the pulmonary circulation, with resultant right heart failure, atelectasis, hypoxaemia, decreased cardiac output or cardiac arrest.

17 **Patients most at risk of developing a deep venous thrombosis are:**

a) post-operative patients   b) ambulatory patients
c) pre-operative patients   d) asthmatic patients

Post-operative patients are at risk of decreased venous return. Consequently, post-operative patients should be provided with compression stockings to prevent venous stasis and thus decrease the risk of developing a deep venous thrombosis. Care must be taken when selecting compression stockings. It is important to ensure that the stocking fits correctly and delivers the correct level of compression to aid venous return. Details of how to measure the leg correctly are provided by the manufacturer of the stocking and it is important that this is adhered to.

FILL IN THE BLANKS

18 **The systolic blood pressure provides information about the status of the heart and great _arteries_.**

Measuring blood pressure provides information on the overall health status of the patient. Systolic blood pressure provides information about the status of the heart and great arteries, while the diastolic pressure provides information on the peripheral vascular resistance. A single blood pressure reading, however, does not provide adequate data from which conclusions can be drawn. A series of blood pressure measurements should be taken.

19 **Blood pressure measurements ate recorded in association with *Korotkoff* sounds.**

These sounds are described as 'K' phases. The systolic, or first, pressure reading occurs with the advent of the first Korotkoff sound. The systolic reading represents the maximal pressure in the aorta following contraction of the left ventricle and is heard as a faint tapping sound.

20 **When measuring blood pressure, the cuff should be inflated until the *radial* pulse can no longer be felt.**

A low systolic pressure may be reported in patients who have an auscultatory gap. This is when the Korotkoff sounds disappear shortly after the systolic pressure is heard, and resume well above what corresponds to the diastolic pressure. About 5% of the population have an auscultatory gap and it is most common in those with hypertension. This error can be avoided if the systolic pressure is first estimated by palpation of the radial artery.

21 **When measuring blood pressure, it is important to use a cuff that covers _80%_ of the circumference of the upper arm.**

Selection of the proper size cuff is important to obtain an accurate blood pressure reading.

22 **The British Hypertension Society recommends that patients who have sustained systolic blood pressure of greater than or equal to _160 mmHg_, or sustained diastolic blood pressure of greater or equal to _100 mmHg_, should be commenced on anti-hypertensive drug treatment.**

Persistent hypertension is a common disease and approximately 30% of people over the age of 50 years are hypertensive.

23 **When a patient has no signs of life, no pulse, or if there is any doubt, start _CPR_ immediately.**

If unsure, do not delay starting cardiopulmonary resuscitation (CPR). Delays in diagnosis of cardiac arrest and starting CPR will affect survival adversely and must be avoided. There is evidence that even trained healthcare staff cannot assess the breathing and pulse sufficiently reliably to confirm cardiac arrest. Agonal breathing (occasional gasps, slow laboured or noisy breathing) is common in the early stages of cardiac arrest and should not be confused as a sign of life/circulation. Starting CPR on a very sick patient with a low cardiac output is unlikely to be harmful and may be beneficial.

24 **The correct hand position for chest compression is in the middle of the lower half of the _sternum_.**

This hand position can be found quickly if you have been taught to 'place the heel of one hand in the centre of the chest with the other hand on top', and your teaching included a demonstration of placing hands in the middle of the lower half of the sternum. The compressions should be delivered as follows:

- depth of 5–6 cm
- rate of 100–120 compressions per minute
- allow the chest to recoil completely after each compression
- take approximately the same amount of compression and relaxation
- minimize any interruptions to chest compressions (hands-off time).

25 **In the case of a collapsed patient who is unresponsive, the patient should be turned on his back and the airway opened using the _head_ tilt and _chin_ lift.**

Establishing a patient airway is always a priority, as inadequate oxygenation and ventilation will almost certainly result in cerebral hypoxia and subsequent brain damage. Use a pocket mask to help you ventilate the lungs. Provide enough volume to produce a visible chest rise. Add supplemental oxygen as soon as possible.

26 **Airway assessment should be performed using the look, listen and _feel_ approach.**

Airway obstruction can be subtle and, according to the UK Resuscitation Council, is often missed by healthcare professionals. The guidelines for assessing airway obstruction are: look for chest and abdominal movements, listen and feel for airflow at the mouth and nose.

8 Neurological assessment skills

INTRODUCTION

Neurological assessment is a set of standard observations that relate to the evaluation of the integrity of an individual's nervous system. These observations consist of: the Glasgow Coma Scale (GCS); pupil size and reaction; limb responses; and vital signs. Nurses need to be able to perform a basic neurological assessment accurately and understand the significance of the findings, as changes can occur rapidly within seconds, minutes or hours, or very slowly over a period of days, weeks, months or years. A thorough understanding of the nervous system is necessary and skills of questioning, measuring and recording should be well developed. Patients in any type of clinical setting may require assessment for a variety of reasons, including falls, unresponsiveness, post-anaesthesia or new admissions. The neurological chart is an important assessment tool that must be recorded correctly and changes responded to appropriately and competently. It enables staff to make repeated, rapid assessments of the neurological status of the patient. The main reason for performing neurological observations is to determine if a patient's neurological condition is improving, stabilizing or deteriorating.

Useful resources

The Royal Marsden Hospital Manual of Clinical Nursing Procedures

Head Injury: Triage, assessment, investigation and early management of head injury in infants, children and adults

Nurses! Test Yourself in Anatomy and Physiology
Chapter 5

Nurses! Test Yourself in Pathophysiology
Chapter 5

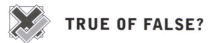

TRUE OF FALSE?

Are the following statements true or false?

1 Neurological function is determined by recording the Glasgow Coma Scale (GCS) and vital signs.

2 Arousability is a state or appearance of being awake that reflects the activity of the reticular activating system (RAS).

3 Awareness refers to the content of consciousness, including cognitive function and reflects the activity of the brainstem.

4 The Glasgow Coma Scale is an internationally recognized tool that assesses a patient's level of consciousness.

5 The Glasgow Coma Scale uses a scoring system based on three areas of assessment: eye opening (maximum score of 4), best verbal response (maximum score of 4) and best motor response (maximum score of 4).

6 Assessment of motor response involves recording the best response of all four limbs.

7 A peripheral stimulus is interpreted via the peripheral nervous system and communicates with the central nervous system via the spinal cord to the brain.

8 Assessment of limb movements provides information about motor function.

9 If a patient 'localizes to pain', he will extend his arms.

10 Pupil size is measured in millimetres.

MULTIPLE CHOICE

Identify one correct answer for each of the following

11 A neurological assessment involves recording:

a) the Glasgow Coma Scale

b) the Glasgow Coma Scale, pupil size and response to light, vital signs

c) the limb responses, Glasgow Coma Scale, pupil size and response to light

d) the Glasgow Coma Scale, pupil size and response to light, limb responses, vital signs

12 The purpose of the Glasgow Coma Scale is:

a) to assess the severity of the patient's injury

b) to measure the level of consciousness

c) to assess the patient's cognitive ability

d) to standardize clinical observations of a head injury patient

13 The specific components of the Glasgow Coma Scale are:

a) eye opening, verbal response, motor response, pupil response, limb movement

b) eye opening, verbal response, pupil response

c) eye opening, pupil response, limb response

d) eye opening, verbal response, motor response

14 Eye opening response indicates:

a) the cerebral cortex is intact

b) the patient is orientated

c) the patient is aware of his surroundings

d) the arousal mechanism in the brain is active

15 On assessment of *verbal response* the patient will score V5 if he is able to answer questions correctly about:

a) name, date of birth, present year

b) date, present location, season

c) full name, present location, current year

d) month, date, full name

16 The most suitable recommended method of applying a central painful stimulus is:

a) sternal rub

b) trapezius muscle squeeze

c) supraorbital ridge pressure

d) jaw angle pressure

17 The National Institute for Health and Clinical Excellence (NICE) recommends that the minimum, acceptable, documented, neurological observations of a patient with a head injury are:

a) Glasgow Coma Scale, respiratory rate, blood oxygen saturation, limb movements

b) blood oxygen saturation, respiratory rate, heart rate, blood pressure, temperature, pupil size and reactivity

c) Glasgow Coma Scale, respiratory rate, heart rate, blood pressure, temperature

d) pupil size and reactivity, Glasgow Coma Scale, limb movements, respiratory rate, heart rate, blood pressure, temperature, blood oxygen saturation

18 A patient with a GCS score of 10/15 could be responding as follows:

a) opening eyes spontaneously, making incomprehensible sounds and obeying commands

b) opening eyes to pain, using inappropriate words and flexing abnormally to pain

c) opening eyes to pain, confused and flexing normally to pain

d) not opening eyes to pain, making incomprehensible sounds and extending to pain

FILL IN THE BLANKS

Fill in the blanks in each statement using the words in the box below.
Not all of them are required, so choose carefully.

confused	extension
spontaneously	central
to pain	coma
flexion	to speech
motor	sensory
dysphagia	intracranial pressure
dysphasia	inappropriate
peripheral	

19 A patient who opens his eyes _____ will score E3.

20 Motor response score M3 indicates that your patient has abnormal _____ to pain.

21 '_____ to pain' is a behaviour demonstrated in the best motor response category score M2.

22 A trapezius muscle squeeze is a _____ painful stimulus.

23 A patient who uses _____ words that do not make sense will score V3.

24 A _____ patient will score V4 when he can hold a conversation with the nurse, but gives inaccurate information.

25 A deterioration of 1 point in the _____ response score is clinically significant and must be reported immediately.

26 An alteration in pupil size, shape or reaction could indicate a rise in _____ _____.

27 If the patient has _____, this should be recorded on the chart with the letter 'D'.

28 A GCS score of <8/15 would indicate the patient is in a _____.

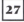

CHART EXERCISES

The following exercise tests your ability to use the Glasgow Coma Scale chart.

29 Record and plot the GCS scores on the chart opposite:

- E4 V5 M6 @ 10.00h
- E4 V4 M6 @ 12.00h
- E3 V4 M6 @ 12.30h
- E2 V2 M5 @ 13.00h
- E2 V2 M3 @ 13.15h
- E1 V1 M1 @ 13.30h

		10.00h	12.00h	12.30h	13.00h	13.15h	13.30h
Eyes open	4						
	3						
	2						
	1						
Best verbal response	5						
	4						
	3						
	2						
	1						
Best motor response	6						
	5						
	4						
	3						
	2						
	1						
Coma score							

30 Calculate the GCS scores and record on the chart.

31 What is the significance of the recordings at 13.15 h and 13.30 h?

LABELLING EXERCISE

| 32–37 | Label the diagram in Figure 8.1, using the terms provided in the box overleaf.

Figure 8.1

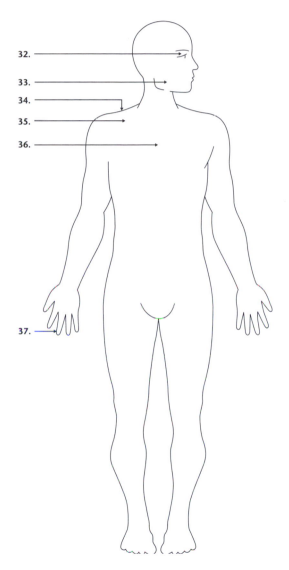

trapezius muscle   central painful stimulus site

supraorbital ridge   peripheral painful stimulus site

sternal rub   jaw margin pressure

MATCH THE TERMS

38–40 Complete the GCS charts below by selecting a category and matching this with the expected response.

38 Eye opening

- To pain
- Eyes open spontaneously without stimulation. Eyes open on approach
- Spontaneous
- Eyes open with painful/noxious stimuli (peripheral)
- To speech

Category	Score	Response
	4	
	3	Eyes open to verbal stimulation (normal, raised or repeated). Light touch on a person's shoulder
	2	
None	1	No eye opening regardless of level of stimulation

39 Best verbal response

- Confused
- Incomprehensible sounds
- Able to answer in sentences using correct language but cannot answer orientation questions appropriately. Responses are incorrect to questions
- No verbal response despite verbal or other stimuli. Does not speak or make sounds at all
- Uses incomprehensible words in a random or disorganized fashion. Expletives. Unsuitable responses

Category	Score	Response
Orientated	5	Able to give accurate information regarding time, place and person. Know who they are, where they are, month and year – not the day or date. Able to use grammatically correct sentences. Do not use questions requiring YES/NO answers
	4	
Inappropriate words	3	
	2	Makes unintelligible sounds, e.g. moans and groans to a physical stimulus
None	1	

40 Best motor response

- Extension
- Withdraws extremity from source of pain – flexes arm at elbow without wrist rotation
- Decerebrate posturing (limbs extended and internally rotated) spontaneously or in response to noxious stimuli
- Abnormal flexion
- Purposeful movement to remove painful stimuli. Person moves hand to site of stimulus. Arms only – best response recorded
- Obeys commands
- Normal flexion

Category	Score	Response
	6	Obeys and can repeat simple commands, e.g. raise arms, stick out tongue
Localizes to pain	5	
	4	
	3	Decorticate posturing (flexion of arms, hyperextension of legs) spontaneously or in response to noxious stimuli
	2	
None	1	No response to noxious stimuli. Flaccid limbs

ANSWERS

TRUE OR FALSE?

1 **Neurological function is determined by recording the Glasgow Coma Scale (GCS) and vital signs.** ✗

A patient's neurological status is determined by observing: level of consciousness, pupillary activity, motor and sensory function, and vital signs. Consciousness is a state of awareness of self and the environment and is dependent upon two distinct components: arousability and awareness. A coma is an altered state of consciousness characterized by an absence of arousal or conscious awareness.

2 **Arousability is a state or appearance of being awake that reflects the activity of the reticular activating system (RAS).** ✓

The RAS is part of the reticular formation, which is a group of interconnected neurons that runs through the brainstem (midbrain, pons and medulla oblongata) and into the thalamus, the relay station to the cerebral cortex (Palmer and Knight 2006). Arousability is the degree to which a person is able to interact with their environment with a quality of vigilance. The ability of a person to open his eyes is a good indication that the patient is not only awake but also aware of his surroundings.

3 **Awareness refers to the content of consciousness, including cognitive function and reflects the activity of the brainstem.** ✗

Awareness reflects the activity of the *cerebral cortex*. The changes in the person will be in their mental and intellectual functions and in their emotional/mood state. There must be interaction between the cerebral cortex and the reticular formation for the individual to be aware (Palmer and Knight 2006).

4 **The Glasgow Coma Scale is an internationally recognized tool that assesses a patient's level of consciousness.** ✓

The GCS has been the gold standard of neurological assessment for trauma patients since its development by Teasdale and Jennett in 1974. It is a practical tool for assessing the depth and duration of impaired consciousness and coma. It was adopted to enhance communication among practitioners to provide a common language to report neurological findings based on observations found at the bedside. The tool was designed to be graphical and easy to use, with high inter-observer reliability.

5 The Glasgow Coma Scale uses a scoring system based on three areas of assessment: eye opening (maximum score of 4), best verbal response (maximum score of 4) and best motor response (maximum score of 4). ✖

Each section of the GCS is given a score and these are summed to give a score ranging from 15 (best) to 3 (worst). Scores are: eye opening – maximum 4; best verbal response – maximum 5; and best motor response – maximum 6. A patient who is fully conscious (i.e. mentally alert, rational, orientated in time, place and person, and able to react to stimuli in an appropriate way) will score 15/15.

6 Assessment of motor response involves recording the best response of all four limbs. ✖

To obtain an accurate picture of brain function, motor response is tested using the upper limbs only. Test both arms using a central painful stimulus and record the best arm response. Responses in the lower limbs reflect spinal function.

7 A peripheral stimulus is interpreted via the peripheral nervous system and communicates with the central nervous system via the spinal cord to the brain. ✔

A peripheral stimulus is interpreted via the peripheral nervous system (spinal nerves) and communicates with the central nervous system via the spinal cord to the brain. However, reflex activity may be the response and this does not provide relevant information for assessment of level of consciousness. Peripheral stimulation involves applying pressure with a pen to the lateral outer aspect of the second or third interphalangeal joint. Place the patient's finger between the assessor's thumb and a pencil or pen. Gradually increase pressure for 10–15 seconds. Because of the risk of bruising, pressure should not be applied to the nail bed. It must be remembered that nail bed pressure is a peripheral stimulus and should only be used to assess limbs that have not moved in response to a central stimulus.

8 Assessment of limb movements provides information about motor function. ✔

Limb movements provide an accurate indication of brain function. Any changes in function may indicate a developing weakness or loss of movement caused by raised intracranial pressure. It is important to assess and record each limb separately. Ask the patient to hold his arms out in front of him and observe for signs of weakness or 'drift'. The patient should also be asked to pull and push against resistance. It is important to compare the left limb with the right limb. Limbs are assessed to determine whether the patient has normal power, mild or severe weakness. A central painful stimulus may need to be applied to determine a response. If no response is elicited, a peripheral painful stimulus needs to be applied to the limbs that have not been seen to move.

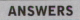

9 | **If a patient 'localizes to pain', he will extend his arms.**

When a central painful stimulus is used to assess a motor response, a patient who 'localizes to pain' will score M5. The patient must move his hand to the point of stimulation, bringing his hand up towards his chin, across the midline, in an obvious attempt to remove the cause of pain. This involves *flexion*. It is important to start with the arm in a 30° flexed position to minimize any anomalies when assessing abnormal flexion or extension (Waterhouse 2005).

10 | **Pupil size is measured in millimetres.**

Pupils are measured against a scale of 1–8 mm or sized as small, medium or large. Normal pupils are spherical, usually at mid-position and have a diameter ranging from 2 to 5 mm. The patient should be examined in a dim light, as bright light affects pupil reaction.

MULTIPLE CHOICE

Correct answers identified in bold italics

11 | **A neurological assessment involves recording:**

a) the Glasgow Coma Scale

b) the Glasgow Coma Scale, pupil size and response to light, vital signs

c) the limb responses, Glasgow Coma Scale, pupil size and response to light

d) *the Glasgow Coma Scale, pupil size and response to light, limb responses, vital signs*

Assessment of neurological function involves consideration of all four areas: the GCS assesses the level of consciousness; pupil changes (reaction, shape or size) indicate compression of the third cranial nerve (oculomotor); limb responses provide details regarding any focal neurological dysfunction; changes in vital signs (respiration, temperature, blood pressure and pulse) occur later and are signs of raised intracranial pressure, which indicates the patient is in danger of cerebral herniation or 'coning'.

12 | **The purpose of the Glasgow Coma Scale is:**

a) to assess the severity of the patient's injury

b) *to measure the level of consciousness*

c) to assess the patient's cognitive ability

d) to standardize clinical observations of a head injury patient

The GCS was originally created to assess the level of impaired consciousness and coma in patients with head injuries. The GCS will not provide enough information about an injury. There are many causes of altered unconsciousness, both intracranial and extracranial, including

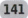

space-occupying lesions, head injury, haemorrhagic events, seizures, epilepsy, infections, degenerative conditions, endocrine-related, drugs, hypoxia, hypoglycaemia and sedative drug overdose. Consciousness is subject to change; it can occur rapidly within seconds, minutes and hours or very slowly, over a period of days or months.

13   The specific components of the Glasgow Coma Scale are:

a) eye opening, verbal response, motor response, pupil response, limb movement

b) eye opening, verbal response, pupil response

c) eye opening, pupil response, limb response

d) *eye opening, verbal response, motor response*

Assessment of level of consciousness using the GCS involves three phases of behaviour: eye opening, verbal response and motor response. *Eye opening* assesses the level of arousal and wakefulness – that is, the function of the brainstem (reticular activating system). *Best verbal response* assesses orientation, communication and awareness of self and the environment. The response demonstrates the integrity of the higher, cognitive and interpretive centres of the brain responsible for speech, comprehension and articulation. *Best motor response* assesses the function of the sensory and motor pathways and gauges the best response to a series of simple commands.

14   Eye opening response indicates:

a) the cerebral cortex is intact

b) the patient is orientated

c) the patient is aware of his surroundings

d) *the arousal mechanism in the brain is active*

Eye opening is indicative of the wakefulness of the patient and shows that the arousal mechanisms located in the brainstem are functioning. Eye opening is a measure of arousal, but does not imply that awareness is present.

15   On assessment of *verbal response* the patient will score V5 if he is able to answer questions correctly about:

a) name, date of birth, present year

b) date, present location, season

c) *full name, present location, current year*

d) month, date, full name

The patient who is orientated should be able to state: who they are (name); where they are and why (in which town or city and name of hospital); and the current year and month.

16 **The most suitable recommended method of applying a central painful stimulus is:**

a) sternal rub   *b) trapezius muscle squeeze*
c) supraorbital ridge pressure   d) jaw angle pressure

The most suitable method is the trapezius muscle squeeze. A sternal rub can cause marked bruising, despite its effectiveness in eliciting a central stimulus, and should not be used. Supraorbital and jaw angle pressure may not be appropriate in suspected or proven facial trauma. Supraorbital pressure is contraindicated in the presence of glaucoma and can also result in bradycardia.

17 **The National Institute for Health and Clinical Excellence recommends that the minimum, acceptable, documented, neurological observations of a patient with a head injury are:**

a) Glasgow Coma Scale, respiratory rate, blood oxygen saturation, limb movements
b) blood oxygen saturation, respiratory rate, heart rate, blood pressure, temperature, pupil size and reactivity
c) Glasgow Coma Scale, respiratory rate, heart rate, blood pressure, temperature
d) *pupil size and reactivity, Glasgow Coma Scale, limb movements, respiratory rate, heart rate, blood pressure, temperature, blood oxygen saturation*

NICE guidelines recommend that if a patient's GCS score deteriorates to below 15, half-hourly observations should be recorded. These should include GCS, pupil size and reactivity, limb movements, respiratory rate, heart rate, blood pressure, temperature and blood oxygen saturation.

18 **A patient with a GCS score of 10/15 could be responding as follows:**

a) opening eyes spontaneously, making incomprehensible sounds and obeying commands
b) opening eyes to pain, using inappropriate words and flexing abnormally to pain
c) *opening eyes to pain, confused and flexing normally to pain*
d) not opening eyes to pain, making incomprehensible sounds and extending to pain

A patient who scores GCS 10/15 could: open his eyes to pain (2 points); be able to hold a conversation, but give confused answers to questions related to time, place and person (4 points); and be flexing normally to a central painful stimulus (4 points). It is recommended that the scores for each of the three sections – eye opening (E), verbal response (V) and motor response (M) should be documented separately to explain exactly which score has been awarded in each category, i.e. E2 V4 M4.

FILL IN THE BLANKS

19 **A patient who opens his eyes *to speech* will score E3.**

It is important to differentiate between a person sleeping and being unresponsive. This can be done by asking the patient to 'open your eyes, please'. It may be necessary to raise your voice until you are sure that there is no response to a loud stimulus.

20 **Motor response score M3 indicates that your patient has abnormal *flexion* to pain.**

Abnormal flexion and extension represent abnormal movements. The terms 'decorticate' and 'decerebrate' rigidity are used. Decorticate rigidity is *abnormal flexion* and occurs when there is a block in the motor pathway between the cerebral cortex and the brainstem. It is a much slower response to a painful stimulus, and can be recognized by the patient flexing his arms and rotating his wrist. The thumb may also flex and move across the fingers.

21 **'*Extension* to pain' is a behaviour demonstrated in the best motor response category score M2.**

Extension to pain is representative of decerebrate activity and reflects disturbance of the midbrain and pons. The patient will straighten his arms and rotate his shoulders inwards. Legs may also straighten with plantar flexion of feet (toes point down).

22 **A trapezius muscle squeeze is a *central* painful stimulus.**

A central stimulus applies noxious painful stimuli to the 'core' of the central nervous system. It is used to assess the integrity of the higher centres of the brain in an area where it is not possible to activate a reflex action response. It is performed by grasping approximately 3 cm of the trapezius muscle between the thumb and forefinger and twisting. The painful stimulus should be applied for a maximum of 30 seconds and it may take up to 20 seconds to elicit the true response.

23 **A patient who uses *inappropriate* words that do not make sense will score V3.**

The patient may be articulating words clearly but he will not be constructing sentences. Words will be random and disorganized. He may be agitated, swearing and at times aggressive. Painful stimuli may be required to elicit a response.

24 A *confused* patient will score V4 when he can hold a conversation with the nurse, but gives inaccurate information.

The patient will be talking in grammatically correct sentences while focusing his attention on the nurse. He may be unable to answer questions related to time, place and person correctly. Questions should refer to current orientation and not to information that may be in his long-term memory.

25 A deterioration of 1 point in the *motor* response score is clinically significant and must be reported immediately.

NICE guidelines (2007) suggest that if any of the following changes in a patient's condition are observed, the patient should be reviewed by a second member of staff who is competent to perform the observation: agitation or abnormal behaviour noted; GCS dropped by 1 point and lasted for at least 30 minutes (give greater weight to a drop of 1 point in the motor response score); any drop of 3 or more points in eye opening or verbal response score, or 2 or more points in the motor response score; severe or increasing headache developed or persistent vomiting; new or evolving neurological symptoms or signs, such as pupil inequality or asymmetry of limb or facial movement.

26 An alteration in pupil size, shape or reaction could indicate a rise in *intracranial pressure*.

Any changes in the patient's pupil reaction, shape or size are a *late* sign of raised intracranial pressure. Sluggish or suddenly dilated unequal pupils are an indication that oedema or haematoma is worsening and the third cranial nerve (oculomotor) is being compressed through the foramen magnum. Pupil reaction to light should be brisk and, after removal of the light source, the pupil should return to its original size. There should be a consensual reaction to the light source – that is, the opposite pupil also constricts when the light source is applied to the other eye.

27 If the patient has *dysphasia*, this should be recorded on the chart with the letter 'D'.

It may not be possible to obtain an accurate score for the verbal response category if a patient has dysphasia, thus a 'D must be recorded. If the patient is unable to open his eyes due to swelling or surgery, a 'C' (for closed) is recorded. Also, if a tracheostomy or endotracheal tube is in situ, use 'T' or 'ET'. Recordings are put in the 'none' column and all reasons clearly documented.

28 A GCS score of <8/15 would indicate the patient is in a *coma*.

A patient with a GCS <8/15 requires urgent medical attention to provide appropriate airway management and resuscitation. It is vital that staff record exactly what is being observed, as changes can be rapid and require an immediate response.

CHART EXERCISES

29 Record and plot the GCS scores on the chart below:

		10.00	12.00	12.30	13.00	13.15	13.30
Eyes open	4						
	3						
	2						
	1						
Best verbal response	5						
	4						
	3						
	2						
	1						
Best motor response	6						
	5						
	4						
	3						
	2						
	1						
Coma score		15	14	13	9	7	3

30 GCS scores = 15, 14, 13, 9, 7, 3.

31 At 13.15 h, a GCS score 7/15 indicates the patient is in a coma and needs urgent medical attention. At 13.30 h, a GCS score 3/15 indicates the patient is unresponsive in all categories and unlikely to survive.

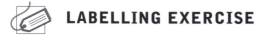

LABELLING EXERCISE

Figure 8.2

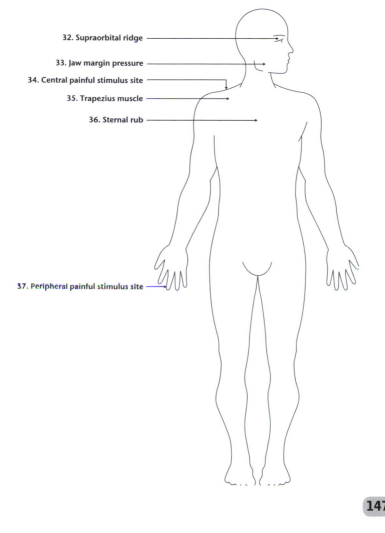

32. Supraorbital ridge

33. Jaw margin pressure

34. Central painful stimulus site

35. Trapezius muscle

36. Sternal rub

37. Peripheral painful stimulus site

MATCH THE TERMS

38 Eye opening

Category	Score	Response
Spontaneous	4	Eyes open spontaneously without stimulation. Eyes open on approach
To speech	3	Eyes open to verbal stimulation (normal, raised or repeated). Light touch on a person's shoulder
To pain	2	Eyes open with painful/noxious stimuli (peripheral)
None	1	No eye opening regardless of level of stimulation

39 Best verbal response

Category	Score	Response
Orientated	5	Able to give accurate information regarding time, place and person. Know who they are, where they are, month and year – not the day or date. Able to use grammatically correct sentences. Do not use questions requiring YES/NO answers
Confused	4	Able to answer in sentences using correct language but cannot answer orientation questions appropriately. Responses are incorrect to questions
Inappropriate words	3	Uses incomprehensible words in a random or disorganized fashion. Expletives. Unsuitable responses
Incomprehensible sounds	2	Makes unintelligible sounds, e.g. moans and groans to a physical stimulus
None	1	No verbal response despite verbal or other stimuli. Does not speak or make sounds at all

40 Best motor response

Category	Score	Response
Obeys commands	6	Obeys and can repeat simple commands, e.g. raise arms, stick out tongue
Localizes to pain	5	Purposeful movement to remove painful stimuli. Person moves hand to site of stimulus. Arms only – best response recorded
Normal flexion	4	Withdraws extremity from source of pain – flexes arm at elbow without wrist rotation
Abnormal flexion	3	Decorticate posturing (flexion of arms, hyperextension of legs) spontaneously or in response to noxious stimuli
Extension	2	Decerebrate posturing (limbs extended and internally rotated) spontaneously or in response to noxious stimuli
None	1	No response to noxious stimuli. Flaccid limbs

REFERENCES AND FURTHER READING

NICE (2007) *Head Injury: Triage, Assessment, Investigation and Early Management of Head Injury in Infants, Children and Adults*. NICE Clinical Guideline #56. London: NICE.

Palmer, R. and Knight, J. (2006) Assessment of altered conscious levels in clinical practice. *British Journal of Nursing* 15(22): 1255–9.

Teasdale, G. and Jennett, B. (1974) Assessment of coma and impaired consciousness: a practical scale. *Lancet* 2(7872): 81–4.

Waterhouse (2005) The Glasgow Coma Scale and other Neurological observations Nursing Standard 19(33) 56–64.

Diabetes mellitus skills

INTRODUCTION

Diabetes mellitus is a common lifelong health condition. In the UK, 2.8 million people are diagnosed with diabetes and another estimated 850,000 who have the condition but do not know it. By 2025, it is estimated that over 4 million people will have diabetes. Most of these cases will be Type 2 diabetes, mainly because of our ageing population and rapidly rising numbers of overweight and obese people. Diabetes is one of the biggest health challenges facing the UK today. Nurses are required to keep their skills and knowledge up to date and have a major responsibility for the ongoing everyday care of a person with diabetes. The skills, for example, include: *administration of medications* – insulin and oral hypoglycaemic drugs; *recording observations* – blood pressure measurement; *examining* – skin, injection sites and feet; *testing* – urine, blood glucose levels and eyesight; *communication* – assessing knowledge, understanding and teaching. This chapter is designed to test your knowledge and clinical skills associated with the key aspects of care of the diabetic person. Each question focuses on one area which you may need to explore further.

Useful resources

NHS Diabetes:
www.diabetes.nhs.uk/safe_use_of_insulin/elearning_course/

Monthly Index Medical Services (MIMS):
www.mims.co.uk

National Institute for Clinical Excellence (NICE):
http://pathways.nice.org.uk/pathways/diabetes

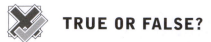 **TRUE OR FALSE?**

Are the following statements true or false?

 Humalog Mix25 is a biphasic insulin.

 Lipohypertrophy is wasting of the subcutaneous tissue.

 Insulin should be injected at a 45° angle into subcutaneous tissue.

 The recommended HbA1c target for people with diabetes is 48–58 mmol/mol.

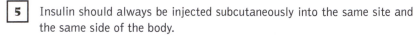 Insulin should always be injected subcutaneously into the same site and the same side of the body.

 A patient experiencing hypoglycaemia should be given a long-acting carbohydrate immediately.

 IM glucagon is administered if the patient is unconscious due to hypoglycaemia.

 Blood glucose test strips can be used with any meters.

9 A blood ketone level below 0.6 mmol/L is normal.

10 A Type 1 diabetic person should be advised to never stop taking their insulin if they become ill and are unable to eat and drink normally.

MULTIPLE CHOICE

Identify one correct answer for each of the following.

11 Diabetes is a disorder of:

a) insulin and glycogen production
b) alpha, beta and delta cell secretion
c) glucose metabolism
d) glucose, fat and protein metabolism

12 The strength of insulin is:

a) 10 units per millilitre
b) 1000 units per millilitre
c) 100 units per millilitre
d) 1 unit per 10 millilitres

13 Insulin syringes are available in the following sizes:

a) 1.0 mL, 10 mL, 50 mL
b) 0.3 mL, 0.5 mL, 1.0 mL
c) 3 mL, 5 mL, 10 mL
d) 0.5 mL, 1.0 mL

14 The main areas of the body for injecting insulin are:

a) arms, thighs and abdomen
b) thighs and abdomen
c) buttocks, abdomen, arms and thighs
d) abdomen and buttocks

15 The rapid-acting analogue insulin NovoRapid has the following profile:

a) onset 30 minutes, peak 2.5–5 hours, duration 8 hours

b) onset 30 minutes, peak 1–4 hours, duration 4–6 hours

c) onset 5–10 minutes, peak 1–3 hours, duration 8 hours

d) onset 10–20 minutes, peak 1–3 hours, duration 3–5 hours

16 Following the attachment of a needle to a reusable insulin injection device, the nurse should:

a) dial up the prescribed dose of insulin plus 2 extra units for the air shot

b) dial up 2 units for the air shot and press the plunger once

c) dial up 2 units for the air shot and press the plunger until insulin is seen at the tip of the needle

d) dial up the prescribed dose of insulin and inject subcutaneously

17 The recommended 'lifted skinfold' or 'pinch up' technique is:

a) pinch up the skin using two fingers, inject the insulin and release before withdrawing the needle

b) lift up a skinfold, inject the insulin and maintain the pinch up for 2 seconds before withdrawing the needle

c) a fold of skin is pinched up between the thumb and index finger and held for 10 seconds while injecting the insulin

d) lift the skin between the thumb and two fingers, and hold until the insulin has been injected and a further 10 seconds have passed

18 A capillary blood glucose sample is obtained from:

a) the side of the fingers

b) the tip of the fingers

c) the side of the thumb and index finger

d) the side and tip of fingers and thumb

FILL IN THE BLANKS

Fill in the blanks in each statement using the words in the box below.
Not all of them are required, so choose carefully.

Gliclazide	monitoring
GlucoGel	hyperglycaemia
neuropathy	glycogen
hypoglycaemia	diabetes
nephropathy	metformin
needles	calibration
lancets	sharps

19 Blood glucose meters must have regular control testing and _____ according to the manufacturer's recommendations.

20 _____ is applied to the buccal mucosa.

21 A patient with a blood glucose level of 20 mmol/L has _____.

22 _____ of shorter length and smaller diameter make injections less painful.

23 Comprehensive foot care is vital for patients with peripheral_____.

24 Microalbuminuria is an early sign of _____ .

25 _____ is the medicine of first choice for overweight Type 2 diabetics.

26 The UK Driver Vehicle Licensing Authority (DVLA) must, by law, be informed when a driver is diagnosed with_____.

27 Put the following steps for injecting insulin into the correct sequence.

	Peter White has Type 1 diabetes and has been prescribed 35 units Humalog Mix25 using a pen device
	Select appropriate needle size and check expiry date
	Pinch up a fold of skin between thumb and two fingers
	Examine and select appropriate subcutaneous injection site
	Dial up 35 units of prescribed insulin
	Withdraw the needle and release pinch up
	Dispose of needle in sharps container
	Wash hands and record time of administration
	Hold pinch up and count for 10 seconds
	Remove outer cover and inner cap of needle
	Push the thumb button in completely and inject insulin slowly
	Insert needle at 90° angle in a quick, smooth movement through the skin
	Collect equipment and ensure all packaging is intact to retain sterility
	Check the prescription and Peter's identification armband
	The injection site should be clean but no special procedure is necessary for skin cleansing
	Wash and dry hands thoroughly and put on non-sterile gloves
	Carry out a 2 unit air shot
	Check the insulin is Humalog Mix25, strength 100 units per millilitre and is in date
	Explain the procedure and gain Peter's consent
	Attach needle to pen device and mix insulin 20 times to ensure even distribution of insulin

ANSWERS

TRUE OR FALSE?

1 **Humalog Mix25 is a biphasic insulin.**

Humalog Mix25 and Humulin M3 are examples of premixed or biphasic insulins. Humalog Mix25 is an analogue mixture of 25% insulin lispro (short-acting) and 75% insulin lispro protamine suspension (slower acting). Humulin M3 is a mixed insulin of 30% soluble insulin and 70% isophane insulin. Biphasic insulins will appear cloudy and must be rolled ten times and inverted ten times (not shaken) until the suspension is evenly cloudy and milky white. The resuspension of cloudy insulin is easier if the insulin is at room temperature. Failure to mix the insulin adequately may result in hypoglycaemic or hyperglycaemic events. Insulin currently in use can be stored at room temperature (<25°C) for a maximum of one month from initial use. It should not be left in direct sunlight or exposed to extreme temperatures. Unopened spare cartridges and pens are best stored in the main body or door of a fridge away from the freezer compartment. Patients should be advised when travelling in a car to use an insulated cool bag or thermos flask and not the glove compartment for storage.

2 **Lipohypertrophy is wasting of the subcutaneous tissue.**

Lipohypertrophy is a benign 'tumour-like' swelling of fatty tissue under the skin at the injection site secondary to subcutaneous insulin injections. When assessing a site suitable for injecting, it should be observed and examined for signs of lipohypertrophy, inflammation, oedema or infection. The swellings should also be palpated. They can be unsightly and painful. Lipohypertrophy can cause erratic absorption of insulin and reduced glycaemic control.

3 **Insulin should be injected at a 45° angle into subcutaneous tissue.**

Insulin should be injected at a 90° angle. The length of the needle will determine the depth of the injection. The most popular lengths are 4 mm, 5 mm, 6 mm and 8 mm. It may be necessary to review the needle length if a patient's weight has changed or because they are getting older. Body fat distribution and skin thickness tend to diminish with age. To prevent possible IM injections when injecting into slim limbs and abdomens, even short needles (4, 5, 6 mm) may warrant use of a lifted skinfold.

4 **The recommended HbA1c target for people with diabetes is 48–58 mmol/mol.**

Circulating blood glucose attaches to the haemoglobin in the red blood cell and can be measured and quantified to give an indication of the average blood glucose concentration over the previous 3 months. A normal HbA1c is 6.5–7.5%. Testing is being standardized and reported in mmol/mol in line with the International Federation of Clinical Chemists' (IFCC) reference method. The new target is set at 48–58 mmol/mol. Nurses need to be aware of this and advise their patients accordingly.

5 **Insulin should always be injected subcutaneously into the same site and the same side of the body.** ✖

Injection sites must be rotated to avoid lipoatrophy and lipohypertrophy. It is important to rotate within a site each day, moving one finger width from the site of the previous injection or alternating from left to right. Absorption varies from site to site, thus an injection at a certain hour should always be given in the same anatomical site. Some people recommend a scheme that involves dividing the injection site into quadrants (or halves for thighs and buttocks). One quadrant per week is used and movement is in the same direction, either clockwise or anti-clockwise.

6 **A patient experiencing hypoglycaemia should be given a long-acting carbohydrate immediately.** ✖

The patient may report symptoms of trembling, sweating, tiredness, difficulty concentrating and hunger. These are mild symptoms and the nurse should treat the patient without delay. The blood glucose level should be tested and recorded. Diabetes UK recommends a practical policy of 'make four the floor', i.e. 4 mmol/L as the lowest acceptable blood glucose level. Patients who are conscious, orientated and able to swallow should be given 15–20 grams of a quick-acting carbohydrate (e.g. 150 mL pure fruit juice or 90–120 mL high glucose energy drink). The blood glucose level should be repeated 10–15 minutes later and when it is above 4 mmol/L, and the patient has recovered, a long-acting carbohydrate should be given (e.g. two biscuits, one slice of bread, 200–300 mL glass of milk or their normal meal if it is due – providing it contains carbohydrate).

7 **IM glucagon is administered if the patient is unconscious due to hypoglycaemia.** ✔

Assessment of the unconscious patient using the ABCDE approach is vital and appropriate action should be taken and conscious level monitored. Management of the hypoglycaemia may include administering 1 mg glucagon IM. This is a hormone produced by the alpha cells of the pancreas. It stimulates glycogenolysis and hepatic glucose output. Glucagon should not be used if the reconstituted solution is not clear and colourless. If the patient does not recover within 10–15 minutes, IV glucose may be required. The patient should not be given any oral treatment due to their unconscious state.

8 **Blood glucose test strips can be used with any meters.** ✖

Test strips are only suitable for use with the manufacturer's designated meter. They must be in date, not exposed to air and not contaminated when handled. The strips must be calibrated with the meter prior to use and internal quality control tests carried out and documented that day. Most of the strips are hydrophilic and filled from the side. The window on the test strip must be completely covered with blood.

9 | **A blood ketone level below 0.6 mmol/L is normal.** ✔

A reading above 0.6 mmol/L is abnormal. If ketone levels are too high, this could indicate the patient is developing diabetic ketoacidosis. This is characterized by hyperglycaemia, osmotic diuresis, metabolic acidosis, glycosuria, ketonuria and dehydration. If the reading is between 0.6 and 1.5 mmol/L and the blood glucose is above 16.7 mmol/L, the nurse should retest the blood glucose and ketones after one hour and every hour while the ketone level is above 1.0.

10 | **A Type 1 diabetic person should be advised to never stop taking their insulin if they become ill and are unable to eat and drink normally.** ✔

The patient will require more insulin, not less. He should be advised to: never stop his insulin or omit doses, even if he is vomiting – often more is needed; check his blood glucose frequently – 4 hourly or more often; check his urine for ketones and if >13 mmol/L or unwell/vomiting – use a ketostix; may need to take extra short-acting insulin if blood glucose >10 mmol/L; if not eating, try soup, ice cream, fruit juice, sugar, honey; always drink plenty of fluids (3 litres in 24 hours) if unable to eat; and take small frequent sugary drinks if hypoglycaemic. The nurse must also advise the patient to contact their G P or diabetic team if they fall ill. Contact should be made if: they are unable to eat or drink and losing fluids due to repeated vomiting or diarrhoea; blood glucose remains over 25 mmol/L despite taking extra insulin; urine tests positive for ketones ++ persistently; feeling drowsy, confused or worried; having troublesome hypoglycaemic episodes.

MULTIPLE CHOICE

Correct answers identified in bold italics

11 | **Diabetes is a disorder of:**

a) insulin and glycogen production
b) alpha, beta and delta cell secretion
c) glucose metabolism
d) *glucose, fat and protein metabolism*

The term diabetes mellitus describes a metabolic disorder of multiple aetiology characterized by chronic hyperglycaemia with disturbances of carbohydrate, protein and fat metabolism resulting from defects in insulin secretion, insulin action or both. There are two main types of diabetes.

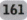

Type 1 usually develops in childhood and adolescence and patients require lifelong insulin injections for survival. Type 2 diabetes usually develops in adulthood and is related to obesity, lack of physical activity and an unhealthy diet. Other categories of diabetes include gestational diabetes, which develops during pregnancy.

12 **The strength of insulin is:**

a) 10 units per millilitre   b) 1000 units per millilitre
c) 100 units per millilitre   d) 1 unit per 10 millilitres

Insulin plays a key role in the regulation of carbohydrate, fat and protein metabolism. It is a polypeptide hormone of complex structure. Insulin is inactivated by gastro-intestinal enzymes, and must therefore be given by injection or by inhalation. Insulin is supplied as 100 units per millilitre. Higher-strength insulin products of 500 units per millilitre are available as licensed products in the USA. The prescription must be written out in full using the term 'units'. Abbreviated forms of unit, such as 'U' or 'IU', can be misread – for example, 10U could be read as 100. Abbreviations should never be used to avoid dosing errors.

13 **Insulin syringes are available in the following sizes:**

a) 1.0 mL, 10 mL, 50 mL   *b) 0.3 mL, 0.5 mL, 1.0 mL*
c) 3 mL, 5 mL, 10 mL   d) 0.5 mL, 1.0 mL

Three sizes are available: 0.3 mL, 0.5 mL, 1.0 mL. The largest of these (1.0 mL) syringes is commonly graduated in major 10 unit markings and minor 2 unit markings. This size is suitable for doses over 50 units. Insulin syringes are unlike standard syringes, as their markings are based on units not volume, and have a capacity of 1 mL or less.

14 **The main areas of the body for injecting insulin are:**

a) arms, thighs and abdomen   b) thighs and abdomen
c) buttocks, abdomen, arms and thighs   d) abdomen and buttocks

The main areas of the body for insulin injections are abdomen, thigh, arms and buttocks. Care must be taken to inject into the subcutaneous layer. The rate of absorption from different sites varies, with absorption most rapid from the abdomen. Absorption is slowest from the thighs and buttocks. The subcutaneous fat layer varies in thickness in the arms, which means that shorter needles (5 mm) can be used without a 'pinch-up' technique. If using the thigh, insulin should be injected under the greater trochanter because the subcutaneous fat thins out down the thigh. The type of insulin prescribed (e.g. human insulin, pre-mixed insulin, insulin analogues) will also determine the absorption rate.

15 **The rapid-acting analogue insulin NovoRapid has the following profile:**

a) onset 30 minutes, peak 2.5–5 hours, duration 8 hours

b) onset 30 minutes, peak 1–4 hours, duration 4–6 hours

c) onset 5–10 minutes, peak 1–3 hours, duration 8 hours

d) onset 10–20 minutes, peak 1–3 hours, duration 3–5 hours

There are five main types of insulin preparations: rapid-acting analogue, short-acting, intermediate-acting, long-acting (including long-acting analogue) and biphasic. It is important to be aware of the onset and duration of action of the insulin in use. NovoRapid, Humalog and Apidra are all rapid-acting insulins and should be injected immediately before or just after eating, as the onset of action is 10–20 minutes following injection. The insulin is a clear, colourless solution and should not be used if discoloured or frosty. These are used in basal-bolus regimes, in combination with intermediate-acting insulin and long-acting analogues, or used in combination with oral hypoglycaemic agents or in insulin pumps.

16 **Following the attachment of a needle to a reusable insulin injection device, the nurse should:**

a) dial up the prescribed dose of insulin plus 2 extra units for the air shot

b) dial up 2 units for the air shot and press the plunger once

c) dial up 2 units for the air shot and press the plunger until insulin is seen at the tip of the needle

d) dial up the prescribed dose of insulin and inject subcutaneously

The air shot ensures the insulin needle is patent and the delivery device is primed and ready to deliver the correct dose. Two units are dialled up and then expelled. If no insulin appears at the tip of the needle, the process needs to be repeated. It may be necessary to change the needle or check the supply of insulin. The prescribed dose can then be dialled up and injected.

17 **The recommended 'lifted skinfold' or 'pinch up' technique is:**

a) pinch up the skin using two fingers, inject the insulin and release before withdrawing the needle

b) lift up a skinfold, inject the insulin and maintain the pinch up for 2 seconds before withdrawing the needle

c) a fold of skin is pinched up between the thumb and index finger and held for 10 seconds while injecting the insulin

d) lift the skin between the thumb and two fingers, and hold until the insulin has been injected and a further 10 seconds have passed

Injecting into a raised skinfold is thought to result in a more diffuse depot of insulin. It is important to lift the dermis and subcutaneous tissue away from the underlying muscle to avoid injecting into the muscle. The lifted skinfold should not be squeezed so tightly that it causes skin blanching or pain. The needle should be kept in the skin for at least 10 seconds after injecting the insulin. This is to reduce leakage and dribbling. If insulin leaks out, release the skinfold before injecting, as pressure from holding the skinfold may force the insulin back along the needle track. Failure to administer the total amount may result in poor glycaemic control and inappropriate dose adjustment. A recent survey indicated participants preferred to use a lifted skinfold when injecting into the abdomen and the thigh, but not for the arms and buttocks.

18 **A capillary blood glucose sample is obtained from:**

a) *the side of the fingers*
b) the tip of the fingers
c) the side of the thumb and index finger
d) the side and tip of fingers and thumb

The side and not the tip of the fingers should be used to obtain a capillary blood glucose sample. The side of the finger is less sensitive than the tip and sensitivity in the tips of the fingers may be lost if used regularly. Frequent use of the index finger and thumb should be avoided, as these are used continuously in apposition. The sampling site should be rotated to avoid infection from multiple sampling and to reduce pain and hardening.

FILL IN THE BLANKS

19 **Blood glucose meters must have regular control testing and _calibration_ according to the manufacturer's recommendations.**

Blood glucose meters are devices to monitor blood glucose levels. The results will be accurate, providing factors that influence the results are taken into account. Inaccuracies are mostly due to: inadequate meter calibration; failure to code correctly; poor meter maintenance; and incorrect user technique. Nurses must demonstrate competence to use the meter and carry out regular control testing and calibration. If the result is thought to be inaccurate, the test should be repeated. If the error persists, the meter should be withdrawn from use and sent to the technician for repair.

20 **_GlucoGel_ is applied to the buccal mucosa.**

If your patient is hypoglycaemic (<4 mmol/L) and unable to eat but is still conscious and able to swallow, squeeze 1.5–2 tubes of GlucoGel into the mouth between the teeth and gums. The outside of the cheeks may be

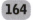

gently massaged. Jam, honey or treacle could be used as an alternative. If the GlucoGel is ineffective, IM glucagon may be prescribed. When the patient recovers, it is important to determine the cause of the hypoglycaemia, which may be: too much glucose-lowering medication (e.g. insulin or tablets); missed or delayed meals; not eating enough; exercise; and excessive alcohol.

21 **A patient with a blood glucose level of 20 mmol/L has** *hyperglycaemia*.

Hyperglycaemia refers to an elevated blood glucose level >10 mmol/L due to a relative or absolute insulin deficiency. The symptoms of hyperglycaemia usually occur when the blood glucose is persistently above 15 mmol/L. A pre-prandial blood glucose is 4–7 mmol/L in adults over 18 years of age. Once the serum blood glucose exceeds the renal threshold of 10–12 mmol/L, glycosuria and polyuria present. Assessment could also identify polydipsia, nocturia, weight loss, electrolyte imbalance, infection and dehydration.

22 ***Needles* of shorter length and smaller diameter make injections less painful.**

Insulin needles have thin walls with wide bores and are coated with silicon lubrication to minimize local trauma. The greater the gauge number, the smaller the diameter. The needles are delicate and prone to bending and even breaking, and should not be reused to avoid pain, bruising and lipohypertrophies. Injection sites should be clean but no special procedure is necessary for skin cleansing. If the skin is visibly dirty, washing of the area is required to decontaminate the skin. If alcohol swabs are used, the alcohol should be fully dried before injecting. Nurses should be aware of local regulations regarding sharps disposal. Used needles should always be discarded directly into an approved sharps container without being re-sheathed. Sharps boxes should always be brought to the bedside. If a patient is injecting his own insulin, the nurse must ask him to discard the needle himself. Under no circumstances should sharps material be disposed of into public rubbish or household refuse system.

23 **Comprehensive foot care is vital for patients with peripheral** *neuropathy.*

Peripheral neuropathy is present in more than 20% Type 1 diabetics after 20 years. It can lead to reduced sensation of pain and pressure in the feet, dry skin, reduced joint mobility, bony deformity and balancing difficulties. Assessment should include: past medical history, type of footwear, social factors, examination of both feet, check that dorsalis pedis and posterior tibial pulses are present, measure the blood glucose level and determine the patient's self-care knowledge. Nurses must check for evidence of callus, discoloration and trauma. Foot care advice should be given and the appropriate referrals made.

24 | Microalbuminuria is an early sign of _nephropathy._

Diabetic nephropathy is the leading cause of end-stage renal disease and therefore it is vital that changes in renal function are identified early. Nurses have a role in screening and detecting changes and educating the patient about appropriate preventative measures. Microalbuminuria reflects abnormally elevated albumin and is the earliest marker of the onset of kidney and cardiovascular damage. It is not detected using routine urine dipsticks. There are several screening methods available, such as the Micral-Test dipstick test (Boehringer Mannheim, GmbH Mannheim, Germany). This is an immunochemically based urinary dipstick used to test for microalbuminuria and can be used in the ward situation. Twelve-hour and 24-hour urine collections are also used to monitor kidney function and detect early kidney damage. The patient should be given written instructions, the correct container used and the specimen must be labelled correctly.

25 | _Metformin_ is the medicine of first choice for overweight Type 2 diabetics.

Type 2 diabetics are usually treated with oral hyopoglycaemic agents. Metformin is the most commonly used biguanide. It acts by increasing the breakdown of glucose at cellular level, increasing the effects of insulin at receptor sites and decreasing hepatic glucose output. Tablets should be administered with meals or immediately after. Side-effects include nausea and/or vomiting and lactic acidosis. Sulphonylureas (e.g. gliclazide) are more likely to cause hypoglycaemia, as their main action is to stimulate the beta cells to produce insulin. Blood glucose should be monitored and the patient educated about the drug's effects and side-effects.

26 | The UK Driver Vehicle Licensing Authority (DVLA) must, by law, be informed when a driver is diagnosed with _diabetes._

The DVLA requires a driver who is receiving treatment with insulin or oral or injected non-insulin medications to be informed (DiabetesUK). Any problems or diabetic complications (e.g. retinopathy) must be reported. Hypoglycaemia is the main danger when driving. All patients should receive education on measures to take, such as checking blood glucose levels before driving, keeping a supply of quick-acting carbohydrate in the car and storage of insulin in a cool place. It is vital the patient is encouraged to attend an annual ophthalmoscopic examination.

27 **Correct sequence for injecting insulin.**

	Peter White has Type 1 diabetes and has been prescribed 35 units Humalog Mix25 using a pen device
1.	Explain the procedure and gain Peter's consent
2.	Collect equipment and ensure all packaging is intact to retain sterility
3.	Wash and dry hands thoroughly and put on non-sterile gloves
4.	Check the prescription and Peter's identification armband
5.	Check the insulin is Humalog Mix25, strength 100 units per millilitre and is in date
6.	Select appropriate needle size and check expiry date
7.	Attach needle to pen device and mix insulin 20 times to ensure even distribution of insulin
8.	Remove outer cover and inner cap of needle
9.	Carry out a 2 unit air shot
10.	Dial up 35 units of prescribed insulin
11.	Examine and select appropriate subcutaneous injection site
12.	The injection site should be clean but no special procedure is necessary for skin cleansing
13.	Pinch up a fold of skin between thumb and two fingers
14.	Insert needle at 90° angle in a quick, smooth movement through the skin
15.	Push the thumb button in completely and inject insulin slowly
16.	Hold pinch up and count for 10 seconds
17.	Withdraw the needle and release pinch up
18.	Dispose of needle in sharps container
19.	Wash hands and record time of administration

10 Physiological early warning systems

INTRODUCTION

Physiological Early Warning systems (PEWS) are increasingly recognized as systems that can help in the early detection of the deteriorating patient. They have been introduced to many healthcare systems in an effort to reduce major incidents and improve patient safety. Although they are a useful guide to the nurse, they cannot and should not replace the professional judgement of the nurse in making a decision regarding a patient's overall well-being.

This chapter will seek to test your knowledge on vital signs and their significance to the patient's condition. You will be introduced to some of the common mistakes made in relation to PEWS and advised of the importance of reporting and consulting with your professional colleagues. The focus will be on the deteriorating patient in the acute setting. although some reference will be made to the use of PEWS in the non-acute setting.

Useful resources

Advanced Life Support

Nurses! Test Yourself in Anatomy and Physiology

Nurses! Test Yourself in Pathophysiology

The DoH Competencies for recognising and responding to acutely ill patients in hospital:
http://www.dh.gov.uk/en/Publicationsandstatistics/Publications/PublicationsPolicyAndGuidance/DH_096989

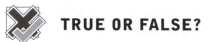 **TRUE OR FALSE?**

Are the following statements true or false?

 In an effort to improve patient safety, physiological early warning systems (PEWS) were introduced within the health service.

 PEWS are only used in the acute setting.

 Many of the adverse incident reports highlight incorrect addition of scores, resulting in failure to call for help, as a factor contributing to the deteriorating patient.

 Immediate assessment, monitoring and treatment using ABCDE is a recognized PEWS.

 AVPU is a PEWS to assess suicide risk.

 In the acute setting, the PEWS always includes respirations, temperature, pulse, and blood pressure.

7 Pain will not alter the vital signs.

8 The normal range of an oral temperature is 36.0–37.5°C.

9 Normal breathing is almost invisible, effortless, quiet, automatic and regular.

10 While PEWS are a useful guide in detecting the deteriorating patient, healthcare professionals must work as part of a team when using PEWS.

MULTIPLE CHOICE

Identify one correct answer for each of the following.

11 A patient who presents with a blood pressure <90/60 and a pulse >100 will have an early warning score (EWS) to:

a) take no further action

b) call the cardiac arrest team

c) take hourly observations

d) seek additional help

12 A useful tool to enhance communication between healthcare professionals from different healthcare backgrounds is:

a) ABCDE

b) AVPU

c) GCS

d) SBAR

13 Communication problems are a factor in:

a) up to 50% of adverse incidents or near miss reports in hospital

b) up to 80% of adverse incidents or near miss reports in hospital

c) up to 30% of adverse incidents or near miss reports in hospital

d) up to 10% of adverse incidents or near miss reports in hospital

14 When providing information using SBAR, the nurse should provide information on assessment using:

a) the nursing process

b) the handover report

c) the medical notes

d) the ABCDE approach

15 The objective of the PEWS in the acute setting is to:

a) treat the ill patient

b) prevent and detect the deteriorating patient

c) assess the patient

d) standardize the assessment of the patient

16 Early warning scoring systems allocate points to the measurement of vital signs. The deteriorating patient is indicated by:

a) decreased early warning score

b) increased early warning score

c) early warning score of 3–5

d) early warning score of 3

17 The key indicator of the deteriorating patient is:

a) altered respiratory rate

b) altered temperature

c) increased urinary output

d) increased fluid intake

18 In cases of airway obstruction the priority is to:

a) administer high-concentration oxygen

b) remove the obstruction

c) administer low-concentration oxygen

d) administer oxygen via nasal specs

19 A rapid assessment of a patient's conscious level is best achieved using:

a) CRT

b) ABCDE

c) AVPU

d) SBAR

20 The most likely electrolyte abnormality to cause cardiac arrhythmias and predisposition to cardiac arrest is:

a) magnesium

b) sodium

c) calcium

d) potassium

FILL IN THE BLANKS

Fill in the blanks in each statement using the words in the box below.
Not all of them are required, so choose carefully.

anaphylaxis	electrical
irregular	width
red	blue
green	yellow
communication	team
decision	leader
deterioration	PEWS
EWS	inaccurate
apex	femoral
regular	SBAR

21 _____ is a severe, life-threatening hypersensitive reaction in the body to a foreign agent.

22 When reading an ECG rhythm strip, consideration should be given to:
  i. the presence of _____ activity
  ii. the ventricular (QRS) rate
  iii. regular or _____ QRS rhythm
  iv. the _____ of the QRS complex.

23 The usual instructions for the application of the ECG electrodes is ____ for the right arm lead, ____ for the left arm lead, and _____ for the leG lead (usually placed on the abdomen or lower chest wall).

24 Non-technical skills are the skills that affect our personal performance. Non-technical skills include _____ skills and _____ working skills.

25 Physiological early warning systems are an aid to _____-making.

26 When managing the deteriorating patient, it is important to have a team _____.

27 Most cardiac arrests are predictable with notable _____ in the vital signs prior to the cardiac arrest.

28 Some hospitals have employed specialist teams to work with staff in conjunction with the _____. These teams are referred to as: Outreach Team, Rapid Response Team and Hospital at Night Team.

29 One of the problems identified with the PEWS is the recording of an _____ EWS despite an accurate recording of the individual vital signs.

30 In the event that you have difficulty locating a peripheral pulse, the _____ pulse should be recorded.

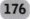

ANSWERS

TRUE OR FALSE?

1 **In an effort to improve patient safety, physiological early warning systems (PEWS) were introduced within the health service.** ✓

Clinical and Social Care Governance (CSCG) is the framework through which health and social services organizations are accountable for continuously improving the quality of their services and safeguarding high standards of care. In an effort to improve the quality of care delivered, CSCG recognized that there was a need for an aid to assist nurses and healthcare professionals to identify the deteriorating patient. The Resuscitation Council argue that in many instances, progressive physiological deterioration occurs over a period of time and 'is either not noticed by staff or is recognised but is poorly treated'. There are specific tools for different patient groups.

2 **PEWS are only used in the acute setting.** ✗

A number of PEWS are available depending on which care setting you are working in. For example, in the acute setting there are 'physiological early warning scores', and the score at which help should be sought is dependent on local policies and protocols. In the mental health setting, there is early intervention and risk assessment tools for suicide, and in child care there are assessment tools to help recognize child abuse.

3 **Many of the adverse incident reports highlight incorrect addition of scores, resulting in failure to call for help, as a factor contributing to the deteriorating patient.** ✓

The responsibility for recording a patient's vial signs and subsequent recording on the PEWS chart rests mainly with the nurse. It is vital that when you are measuring the vital signs that you take your time to record them accurately and total up the final score. Failure to do so may result in you taking the incorrect action in terms of seeking medical assistance.

4 **Immediate assessment, monitoring and treatment using ABCDE is a recognized PEWS.** ✓

The ABCDE approach is a recognized framework in which to assess the deteriorating patient.

A: Airway – obstruction of the upper airway is a medical emergency

B: Breathing – look, listen and feel for evidence of respiratory distress

C: Circulation – cool peripheries and rapid pulse

D: Disability – level of consciousness

E: Exposure – perform a full body examination

5 **AVPU is a PEWS to assess suicide risk.**

AVPU is a scale used to assess the conscious level of a patient.

A: Alert

V: Responds to voice

P: Responds to pain – Get Medical Help

U: Unresponsive – Get Medical Help

6 **In the acute setting, the PEWS always includes respirations, temperature, pulse, and blood pressure.**

These are considered the vital signs, also termed cardinal signs, and reflect the body's physiological status and provide information critical to evaluating homeostatic balance. The term 'vital' is used because the information gathered is the clearest indicator of overall health status. These four 'vital' signs form baseline assessment data necessary for ongoing evaluation of a patient's condition. If the nurse has established the normal range for a patient, deviation can be more easily recognized. Although not a cardinal sign, pain is considered the fifth vital sign and must be assessed at the same time as all other vital signs.

7 **Pain will not alter the vital signs.**

Acute pain leads to sympathetic stimulation, which in turn increases the heart rate, respiratory rate and blood pressure. Chronic pain decreases the pulse rate as a response to parasympathetic stimulation, and may decrease heart rate and respirations.

8 **The normal range of an oral temperature is 36.0–37.5°C.**   ✓

Body temperature may vary according to age (lower for the aged), time of day (lower in the morning and higher in the afternoon and evening), amount of exercise and extremes in the environmental temperature. Electronic thermometers are widely used in hospitals. They have disposable covers, which promote infection control.

9 **Normal breathing is almost invisible, effortless, quiet, automatic and regular.**   ✓

The quality of breathing is important baseline information. The normal rate is 12–20 breaths per minute. When the breathing pattern varies from normal, it is important to carry out a full assessment. If breathing is laboured, noisy or strained, an obstruction may be affecting the breathing pattern, which could lead to a major alteration in the patient's homeostasis. In addition, if the respiratory rate is high (>25 breaths per minute) or increasing, this is indicative of illness and a warning that the patient may deteriorate suddenly.

10 **While PEWS are a useful guide in detecting the deteriorating patient, healthcare professionals must work as part of a team when using PEWS.** ✔

Team work and good communication are paramount to the safety of the patient. The measured vital signs must be shared with other members of the team so that clinical decisions are made by clinical experts who are competent in the specific field of practice and, equally as important, are prepared to admit when additional help is needed.

MULTIPLE CHOICE

Correct answers identified in bold italics

11 **A patient who presents with a blood pressure <90/60 and a pulse >100 will have an early warning system (EWS) to indicate:**

a) take no further action   b) call the cardiac arrest team

c) take hourly observations   ***d) seek additional help***

The patient presenting with a blood pressure <90/60 and a pulse >100 will most likely have a score of >4, indicating the need for medical assistance. The score is dependent on local policies and protocols but you, as a nurse, must be able to interpret vital signs as an indicator of the patient's general physiology and be able to recommend the next stage in their care.

12 **A useful tool to enhance communication between healthcare professionals from different healthcare backgrounds is:**

a) ABCDE   b) AVPU   c) GCS   ***d) SBAR***

SBAR (Situation, Background, Assessment and Recommendation) has been introduced as an assessment tool in an attempt to standardize the type of information that is shared between professions. The underlying philosophy of SBAR is to remind healthcare professionals, from the most junior to the most senior, that the responsibility is on the individual to provide an accurate handover and, based on the vital signs and professional judgement, to make a recommendation as to the next stage of the patient's care.

13 **Communication problems are a factor in:**

a)   up to 50% of adverse incidents or near miss reports in hospital

b)   up to 80% of adverse incidents or near miss reports in hospital

c)   up to 30% of adverse incidents or near miss reports in hospital

d)   up to 10% of adverse incidents or near miss reports in hospital

According to the Resuscitation Council (UK), communication problems are a factor in up to 80% of adverse incidents or near miss reports in hospitals. This failure of communication is also evident when a medical emergency occurs on a ward and a doctor or nurse summons more senior help. The call for help is often suboptimal, with failure by the caller to communicate the seriousness of the situation and to convey the information in a way that informs the recipient of the urgency of the situation. The poor quality of information heightens the anxiety of the person responding to the call, who is then uncertain of the nature of the problem they are about to face.

14 **When providing information using SBAR, the nurse should provide information on assessment using:**

a) the nursing process   b) the handover report   c) the medical notes
d) the ABCDE approach

When handing over information on a patient using SBAR, it is important to include the vital signs based on the ABCDE approach.

- Airway
- Breathing
- Circulation
- Disability
- Exposure
- The early warning score is . . .

This will provide the second party with accurate factual information and assist in decision-making regarding the next stage of treatment for the patient.

15 **The objective of the PEWS in the acute setting is to:**

a) treat the ill patient
b) prevent and detect the deteriorating patient
c) assess the patient
d) standardize the assessment of the patient

The objective of any PEWS is to prevent and detect the deteriorating patient. In the acute setting, the early recognition of the deteriorating patient can prevent cardiorespiratory arrest. According to the Resuscitation Council (UK), early recognition and effective treatment of the deteriorating patient might prevent cardiac arrest, death or an unanticipated intensive care unit (ICU) admission.

16 **Early warning scoring systems allocate points to the measurement of vital signs. The deteriorating patient is indicated by:**

a) decreased early warning score *b) increased early warning score*

c) early warning score of 3–5 d) early warning score of 3

Early warning scores are calculated using a formula that includes an arbitrary agreed normal range for the measurement of routine vital signs. For example, a systolic blood pressure of 101–110 mmHg might be given a score of 1 but a systolic blood pressure of >250 mmHg might also be given a score of 1. The weighted score of one or more vital sign indicates the level of intervention required. The higher the EWS, the more urgent the need for help. An increased score indicates an increased risk of deterioration and death.

17 **The key indicator of the deteriorating patient is:**

a) altered respiratory rate b) altered temperature

c) increased urinary output d) increased fluid intake

Changes to the respiratory rate can often be the first sign that the patient is deteriorating. The normal respiratory rate is 12–20 breaths per minute. A high (>25 breaths per minute) or low (<8 breaths per minute) rate is an indicator of severe illness and a warning that the patient may deteriorate suddenly. When the pattern of respirations is altered, ongoing evaluation yields important clues to a patient's changing condition. Expert help should be sought immediately.

18 **In cases of airway obstruction the priority is to:**

a) administer high-concentration oxygen

b) remove the obstruction

c) administer low-concentration oxygen

d) administer oxygen via nasal specs

The priority is to ensure that the obstructed airway is cleared. This can usually be achieved by airway opening manoeuvres, such as head tilt, chin lift, use of suction, insertion of an oropharyngeal or nasopharyngeal airway. When you are sure the airway is patent, high-flow oxygen using a mask with an oxygen reservoir should be administered. Remember airway obstruction is an emergency!

19 **A rapid assessment of a patient's conscious level is best achieved using:**

a) CRT b) ABCDE *c) AVPU* d) SBAR

According to the Resuscitation Council (UK), the most effective way to make an initial assessment of the patient's conscious level is to use the AVPU method:

- Alert
- Responds to Vocal stimuli
- Responds to Painful stimuli
- Unresponsive to all stimuli

This should take less than 30 seconds and will ensure that your request for additional help is immediate.

20 | **The most likely electrolyte abnormality to cause cardiac arrhythmias and predisposition to cardiac arrest is:**

a) magnesium   b) sodium   c) calcium   **d) potassium**

As a nurse, you must be vigilant to monitor patients' urea and electrolyte results. An abnormal potassium result poses the greatest risk to the patient. There are symptoms you should be aware of that might indicate abnormally high/low potassium levels, including patient complaining of pins and needles sensation and/or generalized weakness. In such cases, you should also order an ECG for the patient and inform the doctor.

FILL IN THE BLANKS

21 | **_Anaphylaxis_ is a severe, life-threatening hypersensitive reaction in the body to a foreign agent.**

Guidelines for anaphylactic reactions resuscitation suggest that anaphylaxis is not always recognized. It can be triggered by a number of things, including food, drugs and venom. Food triggers are most common in children and drug triggers in older people. The ABCDE approach should be used to assess the patient. You should be vigilant for airway problems, as many anaphylactic reactions can cause the throat and tongue to swell, resulting in the patient having difficulty breathing. Breathing can become fast with evidence of confusion due to hypoxia. A tachycardia in conjunction with hypotension is normally also present.

22 | **When reading an ECG rhythm strip, consideration should be given to:**

i. the presence of **_electrical_** activity

ii. the ventricular (QRS) rate

iii. regular or **_irregular_** QRS rhythm

iv. the **_width_** of the QRS complex

The Resuscitation Council (UK) suggests that any cardiac rhythm can be described accurately using these four steps. You will need this information (as part of SBAR) to ensure that the patient is managed safely and effectively.

23 **The usual instructions for the application of the ECG electrodes is _red_ for the right arm lead, _yellow_ for the left arm lead, and _green_ for the leG lead (usually placed on the abdomen or lower chest wall).**

Most leads are colour-coded to help with the correct connection. Make sure the skin is dry and the electrodes should be placed over bone rather than muscle.

24 **Non-technical skills are the skills that affect our personal performance. Non-technical skills include _communication_ skills and _team_ working skills.**

The importance of non-technical skills is now recognized as crucial to reduce adverse incidents in the management of the deteriorating patient. Following an analysis of adverse incidents in anaesthesia, 80% of failures were attributed to non-technical skills such as communication, checking drug doses and planning and team organization. There is much to be learned from this in a nursing context. No health professional can afford to be complacent regarding the importance of non-technical skills.

25 **Physiological early warning systems are an aid to _decision-making_.**

Decision-making is the cognitive process of choosing the correct course of action. As a nurse, you may have recorded an EWS of zero; however, your clinical judgement may be telling you that all is not well with the patient. Clinical judgement is based on experience and should not be ignored. In such circumstances, the best course of action is to consult with another member of the team and then decide on the appropriate action.

26 **When managing the deteriorating patient, it is important to have a team _leader_.**

A team leader provides guidance, direction and instruction to the team members to enable successful completion of their stated objective. The team leader is not always the most senior person; the team leader is someone who is able to delegate tasks appropriately and has sufficient knowledge about the patient's condition. It is not unusual for the team leader to change in the course of managing the situation; for example, when someone more knowledgeable about the patient's condition joins the team, they may assume the leadership role.

27 **Most cardiac arrests are predictable with notable _deterioration_ in the vital signs prior to the cardiac arrest.**

According to the Resuscitation Council (UK), most cardiac arrests in hospital are not sudden or unpredictable events; in approximately 80% of cases, there is deterioration in clinical signs during the first few hours before cardiac arrest. These patients often have slow and progressive physiological deterioration, particularly hypoxia and hypotension (i.e. airway, breathing, circulation problems), that goes unnoticed by staff or is recognized but treated poorly.

28 **Some hospitals have employed specialist teams to work with staff in conjunction with the _PEWS._ These teams are referred to as: Outreach Team, Rapid Response Team and Hospital at Night Team.**

The early warning score (EWS) will help to determine whether the specialist team should be called. All PEWS have criteria regarding the EWS that requires the nurse to call for additional help; the type of help is normally directly related to the EWS. For example, a score of 3–5 might require you to inform the nurse in charge but a score of 7–8 might require you to call one of the specialist teams.

29 **One of the problems identified with the PEWS is the recording of an _inaccurate_ EWS despite an accurate recording of the individual vital signs.**

Despite the relatively simple calculations involved in arriving at the EWS, mistakes are made. It is therefore vitally important that those involved in recording the vital signs are accurate in calculating the final score. Failure to do so will mean that patients who should be referred to receive additional help are not and the results can, on occasions, be catastrophic.

30 **In the event that you have difficulty locating a peripheral pulse, the _apex_ pulse should be recorded.**

Occasionally, the peripheral pulse may be difficult to feel or be irregular. In such cases, the apex pulse should be recorded and the medical staff informed. (This may not affect the EWS but it should be reported.)

Glossary

Albumin: a group of protein substances. They are soluble in water, coaguable by heat, and composed of carbon, hydrogen, nitrogen, oxygen and sulphur.

Allergy: an alteration in biological reactivity initiated by exposure to an allergen (a substance capable of producing an allergy).

Alveoli: small grape-like structures located at the terminus of the bronchioles; the site of gas exchange in the lungs.

Body mass index (BMI): used to determine healthy body weight.

British National Formulary (BNF): a publication that provides essential information on safe and effective medicines for individual patients.

Central nervous system (CNS): one of the two main divisions of the nervous system; refers to the brain and spinal cord.

Cerebellum: small section of the brain located in the posterior region, behind the brainstem; it is responsible for coordinating voluntary muscular activity.

Cerebral cortex: outermost layer of grey matter covering the cerebrum of the brain, controls higher mental activities.

Cerebrum: largest and uppermost section of the brain, divided into two hemispheres, left and right (each is subdivided into four lobes).

Creatinine: end product of creatine (amino acid present in animal tissue, particularly muscle) metabolism, excreted in the urine.

Dermis: skin layer located below the epidermis.

Diabetes: condition arising from the body's inability to control blood glucose levels.

Dysphagia: difficulty swallowing.

Dyspnoea: difficulty breathing.

Embolus: a blood clot that is carried by the bloodstream until it lodges in a blood vessel and obstructs it.

Enzyme: a catalytic substance made from proteins that have specific action in causing a chemical change.

Epidural space: the space between the spinal dura mater and the periosteum lining the canal.

Epiglottis: cartilaginous structure that overhangs the larynx preventing food from entering the respiratory tract.

General Medical Council (GMC): the United Kingdom professional body for doctors.

Gluteus maximus: the largest and most superficial gluteal muscle of the buttock.

Haematemisis: blood in vomit.

Haematocrit: percentage of the blood that contains erythrocytes (red blood cells); normally 45% of the total blood volume.

Haematuria: blood in urine, usually arising from the kidneys.

Haemoglobin: quaternary protein found in red blood cells, it contains iron and is involved in the transport of oxygen by red blood cells.

Haemoptysis: blood that is coughed up.

Hyperglycaemia: excessively high blood glucose (sugar) levels (indicates uncontrolled diabetes).

Hypoglycaemia: low blood glucose (sugar) levels (possibly due to administration or secretion of too much insulin).

Hypokalaemia: low potassium levels in the blood.

Hypothermia: excessively low core body temperature.

Hypoxaemia: low levels of oxygen in the bloodstream.

Hypoxia: low levels of oxygen in the cells.

Intercostal: between the ribs.

Litmus paper: strips that are used to detect the pH of fluids.

Malnutrition: a state of nutrition in which a deficiency, excess or imbalance of energy protein and other nutrients causes measurable adverse effects on tissues/body form and function and clinical outcome.

MUST: malnutrition universal screening tool.

Nasogastric (NG) tube: a tube that is passed via the nose into the stomach; can be used for aspiration purposes or for feeding purposes.

National Institute for Health and Clinical Excellence (NICE): sets standards for healthcare.

Neoplasm: a new growth; can be malignant or benign.

Nursing and Midwifery Council (NMC): the United Kingdom professional body for nursing and midwifery.

Orthopnoea: difficulty breathing when lying down.

Pathogen: any agent capable of producing disease.

Percutaneous endoscopic gastrostomy (PEG) tube: a tube that is inserted into the stomach to provide nutrition.

pH: symbol used to express hydrogen-ion concentration; a pH above 7.0 indicates alkalinity, while a pH below 7.0 indicates acidity. pH 7.0 is neutral.

Pharynx: tubular passageway from the base of the skull to the oesophagus.

Scalenes: muscle located in the neck; aids in respiration, coughing and rotation of neck.

Skeletal muscle: attaches to and covers the bony skeleton. Skeletal muscle fibres are the longest of the muscle type cells, have bands called striations and can be controlled voluntarily.

Sterile water: water that has been subjected to a procedure to render it free of micro-organisms.

Sternomastoids: key muscular landmark in neck; responsible for head and neck flexion.

Trapezius: superficial muscle located in the posterior thorax, responsible for shoulder elevation or 'shrug of the shoulders'.

Venturi mask: oxygen mask designed to deliver a set percentage of oxygen.

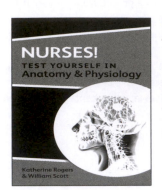

NURSES! TEST YOURSELF IN ANATOMY & PHYSIOLOGY

Katherine Rogers and William Scott

9780335241637 (Paperback)
April 2011

eBook also available

Looking for a quick and effective way to revise and test your knowledge? This handy book is the essential self-test resource for nurses studying basic anatomy & physiology and preparing for exams. This book includes over 450 questions in total, each with fully explained answers.

Key features:

- Organised into body systems chapters
- Includes a range of question types
- Provides a list of clearly explained answers to questions

www.openup.co.uk

OPEN UNIVERSITY PRESS
McGraw - Hill Education

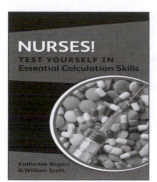

NURSES! TEST YOURSELF IN ESSENTIAL CALCULATION SKILLS

Katherine Rogers and William Scott

9780335243594 (Paperback)
April 2011

eBook also available

Looking for a quick and effective way to revise key points and test your knowledge? Calculation exams can intimidate many nurses. This handy book is designed to help you conquer your fears and strengthen your calculation skills.
It has more than 500 test questions in total.

Key features:

- Provides chapters on the most common drug administrations used in nursing
- Includes quick reference tables of common units, formulae and times tables
- Incorporates chapters on applied clinical calculations including injections, intravenous and paediatric drugs

www.openup.co.uk

OPEN UNIVERSITY PRESS
McGraw · Hill Education

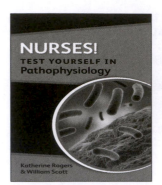

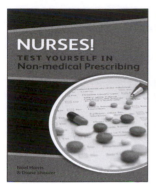

NURSES! TEST YOURSELF IN NON-MEDICAL PRESCRIBING

Noel Harris and Diane Shearer

9780335244997 (Paperback)
August 2012

eBook also available

Part of the '*Nurses! Test yourself in..*' series, this book covers the main topics from non-medical prescribing courses and modules that appear in the exam. This includes pharmacology and calculations as well as the legal, procedural and practical aspects of the prescribing role that are assessed on the course such as: drug safety, consultation skills, adverse drug reactions, concordance, using the BNF and special care groups such as children, pregnant women and mental health clients.

Key features:

- A range of question types, including True or False and Multiple Choice
- Questions based around mini-case scenarios for prescribing
- Provides a list of clearly explained answers to questions, so the book can be used as a 'teach and test' resource

www.openup.co.uk

OPEN UNIVERSITY PRESS
McGraw · Hill Education

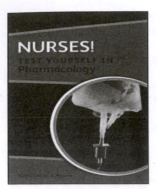

NURSES! TEST YOURSELF IN PHARMACOLOGY

Katherine Rogers

9780335244911 (Paperback)
August 2012

eBook also available

Part of the *'Nurses! Test yourself in..'* series, this book is designed as a revision and study aid for student nurses undertaking their pharmacology module/s and related exam assessment. Containing both self-assessment questions and quizzes, this book will test students learning and help them tackle their knowledge gaps by explaining the answers to all the featured questions.

Key features:

- Organised into body systems chapters
- Includes a range of question types
- Provides a list of clearly explained answers to questions

www.openup.co.uk

OPEN UNIVERSITY PRESS
McGraw - Hill Education

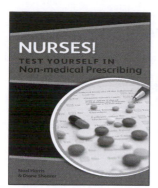

NURSES! TEST YOURSELF IN NON-MEDICAL PRESCRIBING

Noel Harris and Diane Shearer

9780335244997 (Paperback)
August 2012

eBook also available

Part of the *'Nurses! Test yourself in..'* series, this book covers the main topics from non-medical prescribing courses and modules that appear in the exam. This includes pharmacology and calculations as well as the legal, procedural and practical aspects of the prescribing role that are assessed on the course such as: drug safety, consultation skills, adverse drug reactions, concordance, using the BNF and special care groups such as children, pregnant women and mental health clients.

Key features:

- A range of question types, including True or False and Multiple Choice
- Questions based around mini-case scenarios for prescribing
- Provides a list of clearly explained answers to questions, so the book can be used as a 'teach and test' resource

www.openup.co.uk

OPEN UNIVERSITY PRESS
McGraw - Hill Education

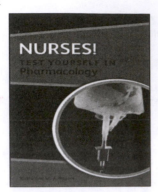

**NURSES! TEST YOURSELF
IN PHARMACOLOGY**

Katherine Rogers

9780335244911 (Paperback)
August 2012

eBook also available

Part of the 'Nurses! Test yourself in..' series, this book is designed as
a revision and study aid for student nurses undertaking their
pharmacology module/s and related exam assessment. Containing
both self-assessment questions and quizzes, this book will test
students learning and help them tackle their knowledge gaps by
explaining the answers to all the featured questions.

Key features:

- Organised into body systems chapters
- Includes a range of question types
- Provides a list of clearly explained answers to questions

www.openup.co.uk

OPEN UNIVERSITY PRESS
McGraw - Hill Education